A New Strategy

FOR THE

War On Cancer

FINALLY!
A New Force Is Entering the Fight
and Its Success Depends on Us

TERRY THOMPSON

NEW YORK

A New Strategy For The War On Cancer

FINALLY! A New Force Is Entering the Fight
and Its Success Depends on Us

by TERRY THOMPSON

The information presented in this book is in no way intended as medical advice or as a substitute for medical counseling. The information should be used in conjunction with the guidance and care of your physician. Your physician should be aware of all medical conditions that you may have, as well as all medications, supplements, and other therapies you are taking.

This copyright is initially represented as a Form TX which is used for dramatic literary works, including fiction, non-fiction, poetry, brochures, reference works, online works, and computer programs. The copyright was formed through Legal Zoom Inc., which has also partnered with VerSign and BBB OnLine. VeriSign is he leading Secure Sockets Layer (SSL) Certificate Authority enabling secure e-commerce and BBB OnLine provides consumer and provider trust regarding resources in business. For more information, address Legal Zoom.com, Inc.

Unless otherwise indications, all quotations, derived concepts, and other data associated with online dating statistics are directly linked to an index and bibliography within the back pages.

No part of this publication may be reproduced or transmitted in any form or by any means, mechanical or electronic, including photocopying and recording, or by any information storage and retrieval system, without permission in writing from author or publisher (except by a reviewer, who may quote brief passages and/or show brief video clips in a review).

Disclaimer: The Publisher and the Author make no representations or warranties with respect to the accuracy or completeness of the contents of this work and specifically disclaim all warranties, including without limitation warranties of fitness for a particular purpose. No warranty may be created or extended by sales or promotional materials. The advice and strategies contained herein may not be suitable for every situation. This work is sold with the understanding that the Publisher is not engaged in rendering legal, accounting, or other professional services. If professional assistance is required, the services of a competent professional person should be sought. Neither the Publisher nor the Author shall be liable for damages arising herefrom. The fact that an organization or website is referred to in this work as a citation and/or a potential source of further information does not mean that the Author or the Publisher endorses the information the organization or website may provide or recommendations it may make. Further, readers should be aware that internet websites listed in this work may have changed or disappeared between when this work was written and when it is read.

ISBN 978-1-60037-777-8 (paperback)

Library of Congress Number: 2010904524

Published by:

MORGAN JAMES PUBLISHING
1225 Franklin Ave. Ste 325
Garden City, NY 11530-1693
Toll Free 800-485-4943
www.MorganJamesPublishing.com

Cover Design by:
3 Dog Design
www.3dogdesign.net

Interior Design by:
Bonnie Bushman
bbushman@bresnan.net

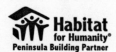

In an effort to support local communities, raise awareness and funds, Morgan James Publishing donates one percent of all book sales for the life of each book to Habitat for Humanity.
Get involved today, visit
www.HelpHabitatForHumanity.org.

*In memory of Connie Thompson
my loving wife and mother of my children
who faced the suffering of cancer
with the same faith and hope
with which she lived life*

ACKNOWLEDGMENTS

To Linda, my wife and best friend, for your encouragement, confidence, and patience as you graciously gave up time and activities with me, so I could be on the computer and telephone researching and writing for this important project. I am also grateful for your companionship on our travels associated with this mission and your help with all of the administrative details. The book is just as much the result of your effort as mine.

To my sons and daughters-in law, Mike and Melinda and Chris and Jayme, who walked with me through the valley of the suffering and death of their mother and mother-in-law from cancer. Your passion for combating this horrendous disease and your zeal for this book have kept me focused through many distractions. Mike and Melinda, your experience from publishing Mike's book, *The Organizational Champion*, and your counsel in choosing a publisher were extremely helpful. Chris and Jayme, your editorial advice from poring over the manuscript for days was critical to getting this message across with excellence.

To my only surviving sibling, Monty, and wife, Janis, who encouraged this work and contributed many hours of proof reading for it. Your sacrificial missionary service in Brazil has been an inspiration to me.

To my friend, Doug Bunger, who meticulously screened the manuscript and provided expert advice and wise counsel. This project is another example of the special events of life that we have shared.

To the team at Morgan James Publishing for believing in my work and understanding the importance of getting it out to the readers. My publisher,

Rick Frishman, invested his years of prolific writing and publishing experience in helping me perfect the book and give it the boost necessary to reveal the new cancer treatment strategy to the public. Lyza Poulin, my author relations manager, always had the answers and made sure I had access to anyone I needed from the company.

To Dr. David Rosenthal, Professor of Medicine at Harvard Medical School and Medical Director of the Leonard P. Zakim Center for Integrative Therapies at Dana-Farber Cancer Institute. Your expertise, guidance, and support at the beginning of this writing project motivated me to pursue the work with abandon. I am sincerely grateful for your affirmation of my work in the writing of the Foreword.

To Dr. William Buchholz, Integrative Oncologist and Founder of the Buchholz Medical Group, you gave me a deeper understanding of the intricacies of complementary therapies that provided essential insight and credibility for my research.

To Dr. Francisco Contreras, Director, President, and Chairman of Oasis of Hope Hospital, for giving your best to my wife's treatment and for expanding my perspective on integrative oncology. Thank you for the interview that stimulated my thinking and added poignant elements to this book.

To Susan Folkman, Ph.D, Professor of Medicine and Director of the Osher Center for Integrative Medicine at the University of California at San Francisco. Your assistance in guiding me through the complexities of integrative oncology research and evaluation was crucial to the validity and success of my writing.

To Myron Wenz, PhD, founder of Sanoviv Medical Institute and USANA Health Sciences, for inviting me to Sanoviv and providing a hands-on encounter with cutting edge integrative medicine. Also, to Tris Conley, Operations Manager for Sanoviv, for graciously hosting my research visit. You helped me see first hand what a first-class integrative medicine facility has to offer.

To Dr. Marie Claudia White for your invaluable personal story of hope and healing as a cancer patient receiving complementary therapies. Your unique view of the holistic approach of integrative treatment allowed me to connect concept and procedure with personal experience.

To Frank Whatley for your inspiring testimony of faith in God and confidence in integrative oncology. Your experience was essential in illustrating the message of this book. Your hospitality and candidness during the interview process made me feel like part of your family.

CONTENTS

FOREWORD

Terry Thompson's "A New Strategy for the War on Cancer" is a book for the general public that presents a vision for an integrated approach to the management of cancer. The author draws on his military experience as well as his personal experience with cancer in his family to formulate a vision for a new strategy to fight the disease. Thompson is not a physician but an academic. He has been quite thorough in his review of the lay and scientific literature as he researched the history of cancer therapies, both proven and unproven.

In doing the research for this book, he interviewed a number of my oncology colleagues and attended several scientific meetings such as the Institute of Medicine summit, February 2009, entitled "Integrative Medicine and the Health of the Public." This meeting brought together more than 600 scientists, academic leaders, policy experts and health practitioners from many disciplines to examine the practice of integrative medicine, its scientific basis and its potential for improving health. In addition, Thompson gained valuable insight from the 6th Annual Meeting of the Society for Integrative Oncology. This society, a non-profit, multidisciplinary organization founded in 2003 by health professionals, is committed to the study and application of complementary therapies and botanicals for cancer patients. It provides a convenient forum for presentation, discussion and peer review of evidence based research and treatment modalities in the discipline known as integrative medicine. The Society makes a clear distinction between "alternative" or unproven and "complementary" or tested useful therapies in cancer care. Integrative oncology is a seamless rapprochement of interventions that benefit cancer patients. The book focuses not on a philosophy of abandonment of the "old" and adoption of the "new and unproven," but on one of collaboration—that is combining the best of Eastern medicine with the best of Western medicine, an "integrative approach."

Following a review of the most recent statistics on the incidence and mortality of the various cancers, the cost of cancer care in dollars and lives and the funding of research, the author then focuses attention on the need for an innovative approach to the disease. He envisions incorporating the evolving discipline of integrative oncology (IO) in the cancer care model. Integrative oncology is to be differentiated from complementary and alternative medicine (CAM), in that it considers the patient as "a whole human being," stressing the importance of all aspects of lifestyle such as nutrition, physical activity, and stress and symptom management. IO emphasizes the importance of the physician-patient relationship.

Since President Nixon's declaration of war on cancer in 1971, the government has invested billions of dollars on the causes of cancer, its prevention and treatment. There has been much progress in reducing the mortality from cancer since the 1970s and more strikingly since 1990. In one study (Jemal et al, 2010), age-standardized death rates for all cancers in United States men increased from 249.3 per 100,000 population in 1970 to 279.8 in 1990 and then decreased to 221.1 in 2006. This was a net decline of 11% from the 1970 rate just before Nixon declared the war and 21% from the 1990 rate, with rates in women declining 6% and 12% respectively. Much of the reduction in cancer death rates seen recently are due to reductions in tobacco use and increased screening that allowed for cancer detection at earlier stages. For some specific cancers, there have been modest to significant improvements due to novel, innovative therapies such as monoclonal antibodies, gene targeted therapies and biologic therapies such as vaccines.

But for many like Thompson, cancer progress has been too slow and often not collaborative but competitive. As a former military officer, he likens the war against cancer to the military campaigns of World War I and World War II, the Korean and Vietnam conflicts and the recent terrorist activities that have killed many. He argues that the old method of "shock and awe" alone doesn't make sense in today's conflicts and our generals seek to propose strategic changes in warfare. He applies this analogy to the war against cancer emphasizing the fact that the old way doesn't always work. Thompson envisions a new strategy of approaching cancer, an integrative approach.

The author has a strong personal incentive for this effort from his own family's experience with cancer, especially his former wife's unsuccessful fight against the disease. He describes the reasons he sought out "alternative therapies." It's important to read and understand the reasons why an intelligent academic professor could be driven away from main stream medicine to seek help with alternative, unproven, unscientific methods of therapy. From the perspective of "alternative practitioners," the author and his ailing wife found compassion and received comfort, allowing for relief of symptoms.

People facing cancer are dramatically affected by the disease, the prognosis and the treatment. Many seek a personal "self help" role in addressing the cancer and turn to the use of CAM. CAM practices are used by the majority of cancer patients and much of it without their oncologist's knowledge. CAM involves some therapies that have now become evidence-based as with acupuncture, nutrition, physical activity, spirituality, meditation and stress reduction, while others remain controversial, such as high doses of antioxidants and the use of laetrile. In some cases, patients turn to "alternative therapies" because they are promised cures, even though these treatments are based on quasi-scientific evidence. Despite new avenues being available for "alternative practitioners" to get funding for clinical trials to test out their unproven therapies, few, if any, attempt to do so. Alternative therapies, including botanicals, herbs, and over-the-counter antioxidants add up to a multibillion dollar industry. Unfortunately, there are some cancer patients that delay a known effective therapy to use an "alternative or unproven" one. The fundamental conclusion posed by Thompson's book is that there are a great many complementary therapies that, when combined with conventional therapies, can improve the outcome, improve the quality of life of the patient and give the individual some sense of participation in the process. That is what integrative oncology is about. As Dr. Ralph Snyderman, emeritus Professor at Duke University, comments, integrative oncology "emphasizes 1) the primacy of the patient provider relationship and the importance of shared decision making and 2) the contribution of the therapeutic encounter itself."

Integrative oncology is an evolving discipline and public attention to the practice of integrative oncology is essential to the successful future of cancer treatment. On the scientific front, new laboratory advances in micro array technology, gene expression and mass spectrometry for proteomics are giving us a better understanding of tumor biology. Soon we will be able to fingerprint an individual's genes and understand their risk for cancer, their sensitivity to various therapies and the best options for control and cure of the cancer. At the same time, we should be incorporating known healthy behaviors that reduce the risk of cancer. As we continue to support the basic sciences, we should be funding more nutritional studies, patient support interventions and doing a better job of educating the public about complementary therapies that support the cancer patient. This book outlines what the public and cancer patients should seek in their cancer care and what they can do. Terry Thompson's goal is to help each individual understand what the new strategy of integrative oncology is about, how to benefit from it and how to support it.

— David S. Rosenthal, M.D.
Medical Director, Leonard P. Zakim Center for Integrative Therapies,
Dana-Farber Cancer Institute
Professor of Medicine, Harvard Medical School
Former President, American Cancer Society

INTRODUCTION

Where Are We in the War on Cancer?

The support cycle for war in our Western culture is an interesting study. A large-scale military response to an egregious confrontation is initially met with patriotic fervor and a willingness to commit whatever is necessary to defeat the enemy. As the campaign continues with mixed results and enormous cost in resources and lives, the citizenry transitions to doubt and frustration. After a while, anti-war sentiments prevail, and there is a hue and cry to completely change strategies or pull out entirely. Until there is a clear victory with internationally accepted surrender documents, as in World Wars I and II, the populous has a low tolerance threshold for protracted war. Do something different, they demand. Either win under the present circumstances or find a new strategy.

However, there is a strange exception to this cultural norm. We are in a war that has been waged for nearly a half century at immeasurable cost in resources and lives with seemingly little hope for victory. Yet, few citizens are demanding a new strategy, and some appear to be more fervent in their support for the long and stale existing strategy as each year passes. Although technology has changed the face of the battlefield for this particular war, the basic strategy and core tactics have remained generally unchanged for decades. A battle is won here, and some ground is gained there; but, by-and-large, we are mired down in a war that has been going on since before most of us were born. The "war on cancer" is a conundrum for our modern society. We would never accept its lack of progress and disastrous consequences in any other type of war.

Susan Estrich, popular author, columnist, and TV commentator wrote a piece in honor of her colleague, Molly Ivins, who died after a long bout with breast cancer. Her words are on the mark regarding the war on cancer. She wrote, "We talk about a war on cancer, but the truth is we're not really fighting one. The loss of 3,000 Americans over the course of the war in Iraq is unacceptable, but losing 41,000 every year to breast cancer is beyond intolerable…We also need to start a new war against the cancers that take our best from us. And this one, we need to win."

Browsing through any major book store or library will bring you into contact with a whole section of publications on alternative medicine. A prominent subcategory of that section will be alternative cancer treatment. Standing in the grocery check out line, we observe that many of the magazines on the rack contain articles about some new hope for eradicating cancer. A breakfast scan of the local paper reveals some new potential breakthrough in cancer therapy almost every day. The upsurge of interest in this subject is because, even though the majority accepts a status quo cancer strategy, a growing sector of our population is frustrated with the lack of progress in fighting the disease. The problem is they don't know what to do about it. Savvy authors are rushing to quench the demand for more information. So, why write yet another book on the subject? Well, with all that is circulating about treatment alternatives, relatively little is being done to legitimately meet the need. These books, articles, and programs mostly proclaim the virtues of their subject, but don't provide a definitive challenge and a scientifically acceptable framework for action. There is an evidenced-based solution to winning the war on cancer, and it's <u>not</u> more of what we have been doing. It's happening now, but it's suppressed in its fledgling stage. A four-decade run of tradition is very difficult to break through.

I need to clarify here that my focus in this book is exclusively on cancer treatment, not cancer prevention. In recent years, considerable advancements have been made in preventing cancer through lifestyle change, various medical tests, and disease awareness. Needless to say, a lot of work remains to be done. Perhaps prevention will be the subject of my next book. But, the war on cancer will not be won until we learn how to get control of cancerous tumors and cells once they have attacked the body. That is the objective of these pages.

Where Have We Been?

The campaign against cancer, although having been fought for many years prior, was officially declared a war by President Nixon in 1971. Since that time, the evil disease has consumed trillions of dollars and millions of lives in the United States alone with little prospect for relief. The war plan depends on a trilogy of conventional medicine: chemotherapy, radiation, and surgery. Although this plan has achieved only limited success, no major changes in strategy are coming out of the war room. The big money and efforts are being poured into improving the weapons systems—more powerful chemicals, more refined targeting, and sharper precision. Even though there is full agreement among the medical elite that cancer is an unconventional enemy, we continue to fight it almost exclusively with conventional warfare.

Unconventional warfare, in the form of complementary and alternative medicine (CAM) cancer treatment options, has been around for decades—some options for centuries. CAM includes both natural, proven therapies applied in conjunction with conventional treatment and unproven therapies applied in place of conventional treatment. What degree of authenticity CAM enjoys comes primarily from low-level research and anecdotal evidence. There has been relatively little major scientific research into its plethora of options. It is like a small renegade military unit reporting decisive wins in a few battles using unsophisticated weapons, but the generals won't acknowledge its successes because they weren't measured and reported in the proper and traditional way. So, the war continues in a stalemate although there is some effort at the highest levels to change the strategy.

The National Center for Complementary and Alternative Medicine (NCCAM) was established within the National Institutes of Health (NIH) in 1999 by congressional law to "conduct and support basic and applied research and research training, the dissemination of health information, and other programs with respect to identifying, investigating and validating complementary and alternative treatment, diagnostic, and prevention modalities, disciplines and systems." They quickly developed a 5-year strategic plan for 2001 – 2005 with goals and objectives in four areas: (1) investing in CAM research, (2) training

CAM investigators, (3) expanding outreach, and (4) facilitating integration while pledging a commitment to practice responsible stewardship.

NCCAM's 2005 – 2009 strategic plan is a continuation of the initial goals and objectives while building on the most successful results and emphasizing areas that have been less successful. The work of the NCCAM in furthering the CAM movement has been praiseworthy. However, much of their effort, including the strategy itself, is like a silo within the vast medical community. That is, most of the activity is contained within the confines of the CAM and integrative medicine arena. The strategy has generated a lot of energy, activity, and substance up and down the hierarchy of CAM evangelists, but has yet to convert the medical science mainstream. A new strategy must take the NCCAM momentum beyond the faithful believers and into the protracted fields of universal medicine. The seed stored in the silos must be sown across the fields before we can expect a crop that will really impact traditional medicine. The new cancer treatment strategy of this book seeks to spread the benefits of CAM and integrative medicine to the entire field of conventional cancer treatment.

Where Should We Be Going?

Many modalities of CAM cancer treatments have been scientifically tested and proven effective in clinical trials. These modalities are being prescribed and practiced by a few dedicated oncologists. The relatively new terms, "integrative medicine" and "integrative health care," refer to the application of tested and proven products and practices most of which were formerly considered to be in the alternative, or unproven, categories of CAM. Such products and practices are finding success as complements to conventional cancer therapies. Therefore, oncologists who study and practice evidenced-based options as complements to their conventional therapies are recognized as **integrative oncologists**. Their practice is **integrative oncology**, and it should be the rule rather than the exception.

Principal areas of integrative oncology cancer treatments include psychology, nutrition, vitamin and mineral supplements, spirituality, physical touch, herbs, unconventional instruments, Eastern medicine, acupuncture, massage, and electromagnetism. Countless testimonies as to the healing nature of various approaches to cancer from these categories are on record. A significant number of those testifying have been cancer-free for many years after being diagnosed in the conventional medical arena as having no hope for recovery. However, too few of these treatments have been given a fair trial in the courts of scientific research. Those that have been proven effective in clinical trials are often withheld from patients by practitioners that remain skeptical. This is due either to the conventional medical community's rejection of their premise or lack of support to promote their widespread use. Those complementary treatments that have been legitimately tested through scientifically acceptable processes are being administered today by integrative oncologists, but only as bit-part players on the stage of conventional medicine stars.

My position is that the traditional strategy to defeat cancer, compared to the mind-boggling advances in other fields of medicine, is powerless. It is ineffective. What if, instead of digital cameras, the photography industry was still trying to sell us on better film and developing processes? What if, instead of DNA, the juries could still only convict on eye witnesses accounts? What if, instead of storing volumes of data on a tiny flash drive, your company was still procuring larger file cabinets? Conventional oncologists must stop limiting their methodologies repertoire to those of the last century. Many more must cross over to integrative oncology.

Well meaning, benevolent people are sacrificially funding cancer research at the rate of hundreds of millions of dollars every year. If not directly from our pockets, we are each contributing to it through our taxes. This money is going almost exclusively toward the development of pharmaceutical chemicals, equipment, programs, and facilities to enhance conventional treatment that is not getting the results needed. Grants and contributions, as well as tax dollars, must be redistributed proportionally with the integrative oncology movement.

Please don't misunderstand me. I am not categorically opposed to conventional medical research. Most integrative oncologists have devoted the first years of their professional lives to conventional medicine with countless successes. Granted, much progress has been made and is being made in early detection, quality of life for cancer patients, and even survivability rates. However, I view the trend toward complementary therapies by integrative oncologists as key to a shift in the overall cancer fighting strategy which can finally bring victory to the protracted war. This trend at least acknowledges the potential of complementary options, proven through the crucible of clinical trials, and put into practice in concert with conventional options. The problem is that the disease is gaining in frequency and strength faster than we can attack it. A cancer treatment transformation of astonishing magnitude must happen, and soon, in order to claim victory over this enemy.

Our current strategy is too institutionalized and narrow to meet the challenge. We must look beyond our present scope and expedite our progress beyond our present rate. We must establish undeniable credence to the prospects of integrative oncology. Our research must extend to include unconventional possibilities. We must make it easier for patients to obtain and afford treatments outside the mainstream. We must generate additional funds to underwrite genuine scientific research in areas supplemental to conventional medicine. To these ends, this book is written.

A Motive Driven by Experience

My objective is to present the current status of cancer treatment, what has to change if we are to win the war, and how you can be a vital part of the solution. I have very deeply instilled personal reasons for this work.

As the Thompson family entered the year 1998, we were on a mountain top. My wife, Connie, and I were enjoying success in my second career as a staff pastor in a large church. Our sons, Mike and Chris, had earned their college degrees, had married wonderful, gorgeous wives, and were enjoying early achievements in their careers. Mike's wife, Melinda, was pregnant with our first grandchild. Life was beautiful. We eagerly awaited that year to unfold. Then all hell broke loose.

Our grandson, Blake, was born with a rare congenital leukemia. He was rushed by helicopter to Arkansas Children's Hospital where he would spend the short month of this life on IVs and monitors. Watching him slip away, day by day, was torture on the parents and grandparents, but was nothing in comparison to the agony that precious little one suffered. Blake only experienced one thing in his life—the evil of cancer.

Melinda was at the hospital with her baby boy 24/7. Her grandmother who had raised her from childhood was also battling cancer. She died while Melinda was miles away with Blake. Her grandmother and grandfather had raised her because, immediately after her birth, her mother died of cancer.

Two months after we buried Blake, my wife of 31 years was diagnosed with breast cancer. The love of my life—healthy, active, spirited, and full of joy—was soon reduced to one who seldom had a good day. Connie suffered through chemotherapy, radiation, and surgeries for three years before her death in 2001. I was, of course, at life's lowest depth at that point. By God's mercy and grace, my children, our extended family, and I made it through those horrendous times, but none of us will ever be the same again.

As I was researching in preparation for this book, my eldest brother, Verl, died of lung cancer. Less than a year later, another brother, Dale, died of a rare cancer that attacked his heart. Neither smoked, and both led healthy, active lifestyles. Their lengthy treatment confined them to the bed most of the time.

My niece, in her early forties, currently strives to raise two teenagers although at times practically immobilized by her treatment for breast cancer. One of my best friends has dealt with cervical cancer for over seven years. She continues in and out of chemotherapy. The vitality, beauty, and strength that characterized these women have given way to constant exhaustion, nausea, hair loss, and feelings of hopelessness. Another of my best friends was recently diagnosed with recurring breast cancer on the fifth anniversary of being declared cancer-free from the first bout.

If you haven't experienced cancer, someone very close to you most assuredly has. It has invaded the very heart of our culture. We must—we absolutely must—find a more promising way to wage this war. It is time to deploy the unconventional forces. Keep the conventional operation going, but open up the battlefield to combatants that are not of the mainstream. Both conventional and unconventional forces fighting side-by-side as one will overwhelm the enemy. And it will be defeated!

Terminology

To get the most from this book, you must know the terms. The cancer lexicon contains an extensive vocabulary. Technical terms are seemingly endless, and even general terms often have overlapping definitions. I have attempted to avoid technical terms throughout this book. That is not always possible, especially when quoting references. There are several commonly used terms to differentiate between the treatment options used by the mainstream medical community and those advocated by supporters of unconventional or complementary approaches. For instance, treatment practices outside the mainstream are described by terms such as: alternative, complementary, integrative, naturopathic, holistic, non-pharmacological, Eastern medicine, and homeopathic. Mainstream treatment is often referred to as: conventional, traditional, standard, orthodox, allopathic, pharmacological, Western medicine, and biomedical. To keep it simple in this book, I will strive to limit the distinctions to just the following few terms as defined officially by the National Cancer Institute (NCI) and other cancer organizations.

Conventional Medicine. A system in which medical doctors and other healthcare professionals (such as nurses, pharmacists, and therapists) treat symptoms and diseases using drugs, radiation, or surgery. Also called Western medicine, mainstream medicine, orthodox medicine, biomedicine, and allopathic medicine.

Alternative Medicine. Practices used instead of standard treatments. They generally are not recognized by the medical community as standard or conventional medical approaches. Alternative medicine includes dietary supplements, mega dose vitamins, herbal preparations, special teas, acupuncture, massage therapy, magnet therapy, spiritual healing, and meditation.

Complementary Medicine. Practices often used to enhance or complement standard treatments. They are generally recognized by the medical community as standard or conventional medical approaches. Complementary medicine may include dietary supplements, mega dose vitamins, herbal preparations, special teas, acupuncture, massage therapy, spiritual healing, and meditation.

Complementary and Alternative Medicine (CAM). Forms of treatment that are used in addition to (complementary) or instead of (alternative) standard treatments. These practices generally are not considered standard medical approaches. Standard treatments go through a long and careful research process to prove they are safe and effective, but less is known about most types of CAM. CAM may include dietary supplements, mega dose vitamins, herbal preparations, special teas, acupuncture, massage therapy, magnet therapy, spiritual healing, and meditation.

Integrative Medicine. Practices that use both conventional and complementary methods. Complementary methods enhance the efficacy and lessen the negative impact of conventional medicine while augmenting the healing ability of the whole person.

Non-pharmacological Therapy. Treatment that does not use drugs.

It is interesting to note that the NCI, a mainstream medical institution, does not recognize alternative medicine except possibly as a complement to conventional medicine. Notice that alternative medicine and complementary medicine are virtually the same except that the former is considered a substitute for the conventional, and the latter is considered a supplement to the conventional. Moreover, when alternative medicine is used in the same phrase with complementary medicine, both become unacceptable. Although, NCI maintains a small CAM department, it considers most practices of CAM generally illegitimate by definition. Integrative medicine has little distinction from complementary medicine—the two are basically synonymous, although integrative medicine emphasizes the whole person. We will refer to these six principal terms as they apply to cancer treatment and avoid the dozens of derivatives that flood the literature today. The new strategy advocated by this book depends largely on evidenced-based research and development of complementary and integrative cancer therapies.

A Personal Challenge

You are about to be exposed to a concentration of information to help you better understand the good and the bad of cancer research and treatment. The book will highlight the prospects for using various complementary treatments without advocating the obvious "quack" methodologies that are out there. It will offer opportunities for you to not only become more knowledgeable of integrative treatments, but to become personally involved. You need to be a player in the critical movement to broaden the horizon of potential solutions. Cancer <u>will</u> touch your life—hopefully indirectly, but likely directly. The knowledge you gain about it, and what you choose to do with that knowledge, will make a huge difference in your response to the disease. It will make a difference in your personal life and in the lives of your closest loved ones. Your knowledge and actions can save or enhance the lives of present and future generations—your children and grandchildren—who will confront the disease. We cannot just keep fighting a losing battle. Now, turn the page, and let's go on a journey of awareness together.

PART 1

THE STATUS
OF THE WAR

CHAPTER 1

THE STATISTICS OF THE WAR

It was seemingly a typical day for airline transportation across America. But, this day was enshrouded in a dark master plan invisible to its thousands of unsuspecting innocent victims. About 1.8 million people were boarding over 27,000 commercial flights destined for important business events, long awaited vacation locations, and family residences. All had become accustomed to the restrictive security measures resulting from 911 and were relatively confident in them. Within a time block of a few minutes, 15 of those flights—huge Boeing 767 jets operated by various airlines—were loading passengers at several locations. These 15 daily flights alone carry about 1.4 million passengers over the United States each year. From coast to coast, some 3800 passengers from every age, race, and background imaginable were embarking on these 15 aircraft on this day. All travelers were busy with their own interests and anticipating their arrivals at selected destinations throughout the country. There were executives with brief cases, families with children, single mothers with babies, and some distinguished elders with canes or in wheel chairs. Pilots and flight attendants in their professional uniforms were scurrying about among those whose lives would soon be submitted to their knowledge and skills. The atmosphere in the terminals and on the tarmacs was as any other day.

Blending in among the passengers and dutiful service persons at some of the nation's major airline terminals were 50 young adult men disguised as typical travelers. They had the credentials and the tickets. Strangely, they didn't fit the terrorist profile. Most were well-dressed and spoke fluent English. None projected a slightest hint of the evil within that drove their purpose. They had been training for years for this day, learning astutely to penetrate the heightened post-911 security posture. Their familiarity with the 767 and airline operations in America had been obtained through a complex network of terrorist training centers. A combination of acting skills and sophisticated counterfeit documents now allowed each of them to board one of the 15 assigned airliners without the least suspicion. Their mission: to kill both pilots in each aircraft and as many flight attendants as necessary, then fly the aircraft into 15 strategically targeted structures that would provide maximum economic disruption. The objective was not necessarily collateral loss of life on the ground, but rather devastating blows to the western world economy. They expected failures, but the partial successes would meet their objective. All that the most powerful and sophisticated government in the world had done to prevent a repeat of such carnage was not even fazing these men.

These particular flights were chosen because they carried the most people, departed nearly simultaneously, and were in the vicinity of their target. About an hour into the flights, the curtain rose on the ghoulish drama in real life. The three or four would-be martyrs on each aircraft commandeered their flight attendants with orchestrated precision using small carry-on items fashioned into weapons. They swiftly began attempting to enter the cockpit using tactics not previously considered by the security experts. Total chaos, noise, screams, blood, and panic were rampant from the cockpit to the back galley of each of the 767s. The skies over the homeland, from the Atlantic to the Pacific, hosted a malady straight from hell. On three of the planes, air marshals with concealed weapons underneath sport jackets dropped all of the killers dead in their tracks within seconds of their initiation of hostilities. On two flights, the terrorists gained entrance to the cockpits only to be met with fatal lead from the 9mm semi-automatics carried by first officers who had been trained and authorized to use deadly weapons. Inspired by the heroes of 911 UA Flight 93, brave passengers on four of the aircraft overpowered the hijackers totally foiling their attack. Although, several passengers and crew members were wounded in all nine of these miraculous saves, the only lives lost were those of the terrorists.

Those on the remaining six flights did not get to end their trauma with celebrations and emotional calls to loved ones. They weren't there for the deluge of invitations for news interviews. They missed the honors lavished on the survivors by their hometowns. Their demise included murdered flight crews, maniacs at the controls whose training was limited to GPS navigation to a predetermined destination, and explosive crashes into key industrial targets. Hours later, after all persons were accounted for, news media reported that approximately 3800 people were aboard the 15 aircraft, some 2300 landed safely although a few with serious injuries, and just over 1500 perished in six crashes. During the ordeal, several fighter jets had been scrambled, but were either too late or didn't get releases to take action. Collateral damage was massive and costs were immeasurable.

Of course, this is fictional—at least at the time of this writing. But is it not plausible? How would we react if it did happen? What if it does happen? The FAA would immediately ground all flying operations, commercial and civil, as in 911. Congress would go into emergency session around the clock. The military and law enforcement agencies would be placed on peak alert. Defense forces would prepare for deployment. The president's hard-line messages of resolve and retaliation would saturate the global airwaves. All ports of entry into our country would be locked down. Over the ensuing days, military and law enforcement recruiters would be overwhelmed with applicants. Older citizens would be volunteering to augment security operations at every level. Old Glory would be flying everywhere, creative bumper stickers would be produced overnight, and slogans of solidarity would be ubiquitous.

Now, somewhat of a stretch but just for illustration, what if a similar terrorist attack the very next day killed another 1500 people? Then, the next day, another 1500. Imagine that for a month, 1500 people died inside our own borders every single day from ruthless acts by terrorist infiltrators. Over 46,000 lives lost in a month to an enemy we didn't understand and couldn't defeat. The most powerful nation in the history of the world helpless against a relatively small group of extremists. Pause and let your mind wander. What would be **your** reaction? Can you possibly comprehend such an atrocity continuing for a year with over a half million deaths? For two years—over a million people killed? Fifteen hundred fathers, mothers, sons, daughters, and close friends cut down every day. Day after day after day.

That is cancer.

That has been cancer for decades.

Within twelve months from the date you are reading this, over 1.4 million Americans will be newly diagnosed with cancer. As you read this, approximately 12 million people are being treated or monitored for cancer in the U.S. Of those, about 560,000 will die within the next year (National Cancer Institute [NCI] 2009). Forty percent of all cancer victims ultimately lose the battle and die. Each day, over 3800 of us Americans enter the battle field of cancer. Each day, over 1500 people die on that battle field. That is the equivalent of six fully loaded 767 jumbo airliners crashing each day killing everyone on board. Six jumbo jet crashes a day!

Expanding our view, we find that, according to the World Health Organization, about 12.3 million people worldwide will develop cancer this year. Of those, 7.6 million will die from the disease—more than 20,000 each day. Globally, 62% of those with cancer will die from the disease compared to 40% in America.

The annual rate of death from cancer in the United States in 1971 was 199 per 100,000 (Steve 2008). The most recent statistics (2006), show that the rate changed only slightly in 35 years—181 per 100,000 (NCI 2008). That is a decrease of only 9 percent over the last 35 years of available record. Granted, we have seen a somewhat larger decrease since the rate peaked in the early 1990s, but the trend still shows relatively little progress over the four decades (see Table 1-1) (NCI 2008). I use the 1971 baseline, because that is when President Richard Nixon officially declared war on cancer as I will discuss shortly.

Table 1-1   U. S. Cancer Mortality Rates

Year	Rate
1971	199
1975	199
1980	207
1985	211
1990	215
1995	210
2000	199
2005	184

Age adjusted deaths per 100,000 population

In over a third-of-a-century following the declaration of war on cancer, American taxpayers have deposited over $70 billion in the National Cancer Institute (NCI) in the fight against the disease (The Economist 2004). This investment, however, pales in the light of what has been spent by drug companies, educational institutions, charities, and other government agencies. All totaled, Americans have spent, through taxes, donations, and private research and development, over $200 billion, inflation-adjusted, to wage this war since 1971 (Fortune Magazine 2004). Yet, all that money and effort over all those years have reduced deaths from cancer by only 9 percent.

Another statistic that has to be considered is the actual number of deaths from cancer. Because of our country's population growth each year, even with the small downward trend in the cancer mortality rate (deaths per 100,000), the total number of deaths from the disease has maintained an upward trend. When the 2004 data was released by the NCI in 2007, the cancer fighting organizations raved about how the declining mortality rate over the past decade had produced actual decreases in the total number of cancer deaths two years in a row. In other words, this death rate had declined more than the accompanying population rate had increased. Although the death rate declined slightly again in 2005, the actual number of cancer deaths increased again from 2004 to 2005 according to the

National Center for Health Statistics (NCHS). So, with few exceptions, total cancer deaths continue to rise each year.

A Declaration of War

As the twentieth century reached its half-way point, the discoveries of new types of cancer and the increased emphasis on cancer registries generated a greater awareness of the disease. Lung cancer in particular was growing out of control. So dominant was the nation's concern about it, President Nixon made it one of his principal goals outlined in his State of the Union speech on January 22, 1971.

> "I will ask for an appropriation of an extra $100 million to launch an intensive campaign to find a cure for cancer, and I will ask later for whatever additional funds can effectively be used. The time has come in America when the same kind of concentrated effort that split the atom and took man to the moon should be turned toward conquering this dread disease. Let us make a total national commitment to achieve this goal. America has long been the wealthiest nation in the world. Now it is time we became the healthiest nation in the world."

On that evening, our great nation became officially committed to the annihilation of this enemy. The president's declaration was later described as the beginning of the "war on cancer." It was to be pursued with the same national determination that led us into the nuclear age and that put a man on the moon. Virtually unlimited resources were pledged.

On December 23, 1971, fueled by the aggressive support of the president and numerous other political leaders, the National Cancer Act was signed into law. This government action infused unprecedented dollars and authority into the NCI to oversee a National Cancer Program of research and education. The NCI budget would bypass the traditional scrutiny of its parent organization, the National Institutes of Health (NIH), and would be submitted directly to the president. The Act funded new research centers and contracted with prominent existing centers in an all-out national crusade to conquer cancer.

This bold venture was not without precedents. The President had alluded to what the ingenuity and power of America had proven capable of producing. We had models of what national determination with enough funds could do.

Nuclear fission/fusion was just being studied by the United States when the Second World War began in 1939. Fearful that Nazi Germany was developing a nuclear weapon, our nation assembled our best scientists complemented by some international experts displaced from Europe. This team, supported by every material and financial resource they needed, crafted and tested a device inconceivable in the minds of previous war strategists. Six years after a concept discussion among a few scientists, an atomic bomb was dropped on Hiroshima. The war against Japan was over.

Sixteen years later, we embarked on another journey of seemingly impossible proportion. Responding to the Soviet's launching of Yuri Gagarin into space orbit on April 2, 1961, President Kennedy boldly challenged Congress and the nation on May 25, 1961, to land a man on the moon by the decade's end. Space became the battle ground of the cold war. On July 20, 1969, just eight years later, the world watched Neil Armstrong make his "giant leap for mankind" to the surface of the moon further preserving our freedom through the aerospace realm.

Both of these historical feats combined cost this nation less than what we are currently spending **each year** on cancer research and education. In the nuclear and space races, the enemy's objectives were thwarted in relatively short order. In the cancer race, we are in a seemingly endless marathon, and the enemy is winning.

CHAPTER 2

THE FINANCING OF THE WAR

Established by the U.S. Congress in 1937, the NCI became the pre-eminent cancer research organization when President Nixon signed the National Cancer Act. The Act gave the NCI the mandate to engage in government sponsored cancer research into the causes, prevention, diagnosis, and treatment of cancer. The federally-funded NCI, operating virtually independently although under its parent organization, the NIH, has evolved into the largest provider of funds for cancer research in the world.

The fiscal year 2010 budget proposal for the NCI was $5.1 billion (NCI 2010). This budget has increased more than 50% in the last decade. Out of its 2008, $4.8 budget, the Institute spent $3.1 billion on research grants, $.7 billion on in-house research, $.6 billion on program development, and $.4 billion on administration (NCI 2010).

The American Cancer Society (ACS) is a non-government institution that receives most of its funds through donations from major fundraising projects. In 2008, one in every 100 Americans participated in Relay for Life events in over 5,000 communities. During the year, these runners and walkers, representing loved ones affected by cancer, contributed $409 million to the ACS. Random contributions from across the United States totaled $270 million. Walk-a-thons, sponsored by Making Strides Against Breast Cancer, brought in over $60 million. ACS sponsored special events and memorials added another $238 million to their budget revenues (ACS 2010). All totaled, the ACS received $1.08 billion in public support, grants, gains, and investments in 2008. During that year, the Society spent $756 million on research grants, prevention and detection programs, and patient support (ACS 2009). About $285 million was allocated to management and general services, fundraising, and purchases and investments.

These flagship institutions manage most of the billions of dollars that are collected and funneled into the hundreds of research programs and medical institutions each year. Whether from taxes paid or donations volunteered, each and every one of us shares in providing both institutions well over $6 billion annually year after year. Of course, there are many other national and local charities that raise the total price of the war on cancer far above that amount.

After the big two just described, the Susan G. Komen Breast Cancer Foundation is the next largest and most prominent provider of funds for cancer research. Focused solely on one type of the disease, breast cancer, the Komen Foundation has invested almost a billion dollars in the cause since it was formed (Komen 2007). Most of the funds come from participants in the Race for the Cure.

Astronomical sums of money from prominent philanthropists are being poured into cancer research centers. One such person is Sidney Kimmel, an apparel industry icon who is probably the largest individual contributor to cancer research. Following his $125 million donation to establish the Sidney Kimmel Cancer Center at Johns Hopkins, he contributed $25 million to the Memorial Sloan-Kettering Cancer Center. More recently, he appeared on the unprecedented three-network *Stand Up for Cancer* telethon to announce another $25 million donation.

Another example of extraordinary individual funding effort is shipping tycoon Daniel Ludwig who died in 1992 after creating the Ludwig Institute. The Institute gave $120 million in 2008 to be divided among several cancer research centers. To date, Mr. Ludwig's generosity has been responsible for cancer research efforts totaling over $1.3 billion (Ludwig 2007).

Not only are national level government and civic organizations enlisting as major financiers in the cancer war. Individual states and some communities are implementing their own programs. Citizens of the state of Texas, for instance, voted to spend $3 billion over a ten year period in the state's quest to become a global leader in cancer research. Prompted by the death of former Governor Ann Richards, the Texas legislature enacted a budget of $300 million per year to be invested in the research. The state effort would be in partnership with the Komen Breast Cancer Foundation , the Lance Armstrong Foundation, The University of Texas M. D. Anderson Cancer Center, along with other medical and funding institutions, all of which are located in Texas (Associated Press [AP] 2007). The first wave of these funds were granted to Texas research institutions just before this book went to press.

Cancer fundraising has become a national pastime. It is integrated into our very culture. Seemingly almost every occasion for social outlet has a "proceeds to benefit cancer research" attached to it. And, who has not made an impulse purchase because it had a pink ribbon associated with it? Some methods are as bland as contributing profits from premium priced postage stamps. Others are as bizarre as peddling calendars featuring nude men or women baring it all in the name of cancer research. Whether we are running shoulder to shoulder with a thousand others in a 10K or dropping our loose change in a can at a fast food restaurant, we are touched almost every day by the constant beckoning to donate a part of ourselves to fight the war on cancer.

This pervasive public and private effort to fund this war is presented as a backdrop for the premise of this book. The magnitude of the "cancer economy" should be considered with every point addressed in the succeeding chapters. Please don't misunderstand me. I am in no way critical of the institutional fundraising. If we are to ever raise the flag of victory over this diabolical disease, it will take even more than the present level of national and international fiscal willpower. The issue is not the money we are raising. The issue is how we are spending it.

Absence of Allocations to Other Opportunities

The billions of dollars being continually funneled into the nearly 40-year-old war on cancer is confined to a relatively limited realm of research and medical services. Very little outside of traditional research and treatment has ever been seriously considered as worthy of these funds. Since the 1950s, when a cure for cancer became a national debate, virtually all efforts have been concentrated on discovering better chemotherapy, radiation and surgery techniques. Most of the medical community has embraced these options as the only hope. Conventional treatment successes over the years have increased quality of life for cancer patients and have brought us closer to understanding the disease. Unfortunately, those successes have not increased the survival rates significantly. Real hope must lie in more than the limited successes that conventional treatment has produced. Real hope will come with substantially more resources directed toward Complementary and Alternative Medicine (CAM) research, and that isn't happening. The objective of CAM research and practice is not to replace conventional medicine, but to enhance it, reduce its harmful effects, and shorten its duration. This concept of complementing conventional cancer treatment with natural, non-toxic therapies that strengthen the body and mind is commonly called **integrative oncology**.

The NCI office that coordinates CAM funding for cancer research is its Office of Cancer Complementary and Alternative Medicine (OCCAM). Out of a 2008 NCI research budget of $3.8 billion, OCCAM reported NCI expenditures of $122 million for CAM cancer projects (NCI 2010). That is approximately 3% of our federal tax contributions to the NCI budget going for CAM cancer research, and about 97% spent on conventional cancer research.

According to their website data, the NIH funded a total of $20.4 billion worth of medical research projects in 2008. Cancer research, including that of NCI, was allotted $5.6 billion of that or 27%. NIH has its own CAM office, the National Center for Complementary and Alternative Medicine (NCCAM). The scope of NCCAM includes complementary and alternative medicine research for all medical conditions, not just cancer. Their 2008 research budget was $122 million, one-half of 1% of the total NIH research grants of $20.4 billion.

Although NCCAM sponsors a few cancer grants and research projects, those projects are minimal compared to the many projects relating to other diseases. So, NCCAM funding for complementary and alternative medicine research gets .5% of the federal budget allocation to NIH, and complementary cancer therapy research gets only a small portion of that .5%. Compare this to the research for conventional cancer treatment that gets over a quarter of the huge NIH budget.

In 2008, the ACS had 10 CAM-related grants in effect totaling $5.6 million. This is about 1% of the total amount of grants being allocated by the ACS to all cancer research and study projects (Sampson, ACS 2010).

Due to broad definitions and some overlapping of categories, it is difficult to determine precisely what percentage of combined NIH, NCI, and ACS research grants support CAM cancer projects. My best estimate is that CAM cancer research receives only about 1% of all cancer research grants. Now, I ask you to pause here for a moment and digest that figure. Place it firmly and permanently in your mind. As you continue to read this book, keep as a mental backdrop the fact that, from its three top investment sources for cancer research, our nation allocates about 99% to conventional and about 1% to CAM or the advancement of integrative oncology.

Considering the meager amount of funding for CAM research, it is amazing how much it has advanced cancer treatment. Studies have proven the efficacy of many complementary therapies such as acupuncture, nutrition, physical activity, spirituality, meditation and stress reduction, and hyperthermia. Think of what could be done with 20% or even 10% of the total NIH, NCI, and ACS research allocation.

The Komen Foundation seeks to empower people by giving them a forum and an avenue for personal involvement in the cancer fight. The Foundation's intentions are commendable as they provide opportunities across the country for individuals to participate in fundraising activities, usually in the name of someone who has suffered with the disease. In the 2009 records reviewed, only 4 out of 92 research projects and studies had anything to do with potential complementary treatment methods. The CAM-related research grants received just over $1 million of the $60 million allocated for all projects. That is less than 2% of all monies raised by Komen activities go toward CAM research. The Foundation implies that it has been instrumental in many cancer research breakthroughs. Yet, Nancy Brinker, founder of this advocacy group, recently admitted, "There is a Great Divide between discovery and delivery...when we celebrate as 'breakthroughs' treatments that cost $50,000 and that extended life, at most, a few months! This is progress?" (The Boston Globe 2007)

The huge amount of contributions by small organizations and individuals are hardly ever sources for advances in anything outside of conventional treatment. Hundreds of millions in celebrity dollars pledged to the *Stand Up for Cancer* telethon mentioned previously were mostly invested in a blue ribbon "dream team" of prominent medical scientists who are to streamline the research process through interdisciplinary cooperation. This objective is highly commendable and is certainly worthy of support. However, not one "dream team" scientist has any background or connection other than within the conventional medical establishment. All donations will most likely support the search for a better chemical or molecular biological process.

The highly ambitious Texas initiative is a welcomed entry into the war. The fund's brainchild, Cathy Bonner, an influential political insider, said the projects funded could change the world (AP 2007). I applaud Texas for its commitment to curing cancer. However, the Texas-based receiving institutions involved are almost entirely focused on conventional methods that haven't changed the world very much over the years and probably won't with another $3 billion.

The enormous amount of money that has been infused into cancer research over the recent decades is mind-numbing. Granted, some of it has funded prevention projects that have helped to reduce the number of cancer victims. Some has been earmarked for modernization of equipment, facilities, and analytical systems. Some has gone for scholastic research. But, most of the funds have the ultimate objective of pursuing a cure for cancer with chemicals, radiation, and surgery. Of course, good has come out of efforts to advance conventional medicine, and we should all be grateful for any advancement. Insights into genetic technology, highly improved screening systems, deeper understanding of the malignant cell, less intrusive surgery, radiation accuracy, and better chemical compatibility and synergy are just a few of the major advances from conventional research. However, the issue is that these breakthroughs have not produced anything close to a cure or even an appreciable decrease in the mortality rate. Yet, every year, increasingly more money is collected from taxes and donations to be poured into seemingly bottomless pockets of those on a seemingly endless search. And hardly any of it is being directed to potential opportunities outside the venues of conventional medicine.

The cause of relatively miniscule funding for CAM cancer research is not totally the reluctance of the funding agencies to sponsor the projects. Research grants are the result of an elaborate application and justification process. The universities and other scientific institutions are not inclined to apply for many CAM-related research grants. CAM research is seen as not being on the leading edge of medical science and has a less appealing monetary rate of return on the sponsoring organization's time and investment. I would like to see more influence and incentives from the funding agencies to encourage the research institutes in CAM-related research. However, little change is likely until there is a groundswell of demand from the grass roots for CAM research.

Many Researchers, New Ground, No Resources

So, if the conventional approach to cancer treatment is not producing positive results fast enough, why is medical science not directing its energies and intelligence toward a change of strategy? The fact is that those operating where the rubber meets the road are advocating change. Researchers want to make something better for the physicians. Physicians want to provide something better for their patients. But, the environment of institutionalized medicine is not conducive to change. The American health industry has been building for years to become the world leader in its field. Millions of people benefit daily from its immeasurable successes, although many are victims of its inattention to their particular needs. Regrettably, the growth of any such industry generates a bureaucracy that is resistant to change. Like an obese person who can't alter his diet regardless of what his body is telling him, the medical science bureaucracy does not change easily regardless of the urgency and the evidence.

Therefore, a cultural barrier exists between the hands-on medical science community (those who do the research and treat the patients) and institutionalized medicine (regulatory agencies, pharmaceutical corporations, medical centers, and grant organizations). This conclusion is supported by a survey project presented at the 2005 convention of the Society for Integrative Oncology. The "Survey of Cancer Researchers and Practitioners Regarding Complementary and Alternative Medicine" by Dr. Oluwadamilola Olaku and others included 321 respondents from a wide spectrum of oncology labs and clinics (Olaku, et al. 2005). Ironically, the survey was sponsored by the National Cancer Institute which does relatively little in the CAM and integrative oncology arena. Generally, the researchers and practitioners agreed that there was great promise in the following areas of CAM:

Pharmacologic and biologic treatment

Nutritional therapeutics

Mind-body interventions

Alternative medical systems

Of the researchers surveyed, 83% expressed interest in collaborating with CAM practitioners. Ninety-six percent of the CAM practitioners were interested in collaborating with cancer researchers. Evidently, there is a groundswell of interest among hands-on researchers and practitioners to charge forward in exploring the vast potential of integrative oncology.

When asked what they saw as the most significant obstacle to CAM research and practice, the single factor most frequently identified was lack of funds (Figure 2-1 and Figure 2-2). Lack of time was also given as a significant obstacle. Time allotted to projects and services is, of course, determined by priorities, which are determined by funds. It is interesting that a negative perception of peers and difficulty with grant requirements were also highlighted as obstacles. Indications are that the brightest and most talented of our medical community are finding it extremely difficult to break through the establishment for support of much of anything outside the parameters of conventional medicine.

Figure 2-1   Most Significant Obstacles Related to CAM Research
(Researchers)

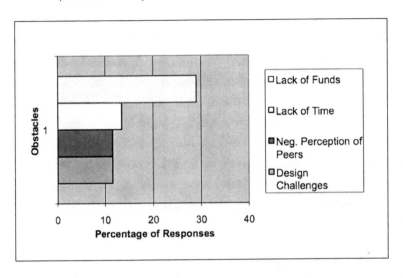

Figure 2-2   Most Significant Obstacles Related to CAM Research
(Practitioners)

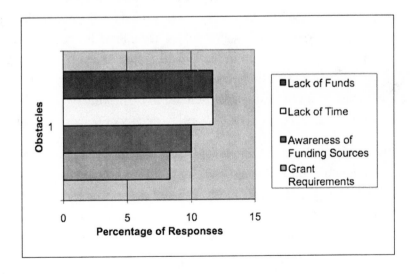

Purchases of CAM Exceed Those of Conventional Medicine

Millions of patients are so convinced of the efficacy of CAM that they are taking advantage of it, often in spite of their physicians' advice. A 2004 NCCAM report found that, at any given time, 36% of adults in the U.S. are using some form of CAM. The National Academy of Sciences (NAS) released a ground-breaking report in 2005 entitled *Complementary and Alternative Medicine in the United States*. This report, sponsored by the Institute of Medicine, revealed that the total number of visits to CAM providers had increased by 47% from 1990 to 1997. The visits to CAM providers in 1997 totaled 629 million which far exceeded the total number of visits to all primary care physicians (386 million). The decade of the 1990's saw a phenomenal movement toward dependence on CAM for all kinds of illnesses including cancer. This trend appears to be continuing.

Further, the NAS report noted that people are shifting their trust away from conventional medicine and toward complementary and alternative practices. Most are choosing CAM in addition to their prescribed treatments and medicines. This is even more astounding considering that almost none of the CAM provider services are covered by health insurance. Shamefully, insurance companies do not generally recognize CAM as a legitimate candidate for coverage. Total out of pocket costs for CAM therapies were conservatively estimated in the report to be $27 billion per year (that is with a "b"). That amount is about the same as is spent on all physician services in the United States. During this period, use of herbal remedies increased by 380%, and high-dose vitamin use increased by 130%. Less than 40% of CAM users disclosed to their primary physicians that they were using such therapies (The National Academy of Sciences 2005).

A 2007 study by the U.S. Centers for Disease Control and Prevention found that one in nine children and teens used some form of alternative medicine in the month preceding a survey. Options included acupuncture, meditation, and chiropractic care, although the leading choices among those under 18 were herbals. Vitamins and mineral supplements were not counted in the survey.

The fact that most CAM users do not discuss their supplemental practices with their physicians is troublesome. Combining certain CAM and conventional treatments can sometimes at best offset the benefits of either or at worst cause grave physical consequences. For this reason alone, physicians and patients alike must be educated and trained in CAM. Oncologists must begin giving more attention to integrative options as an essential part of the new strategy for the war on cancer.

People are using more complementary and alternative medicines and therapies than conventional physician services for all physical ailments. They are spending about as much or more for these services as they spend on conventional doctor and hospital visits. Yet, the conventional medical and pharmaceutical professionals and institutions are paying insufficient attention to anything outside their traditional realm. We have two philosophies of medicine that each have a lot to offer Americans who are suffering—philosophies that should be working together more effectively. Cooperation between advocates of these two philosophies is in the best interest of everyone. The war on cancer depends on this cooperation. When we follow the money, it is obvious that there is not enough pressure being placed on the health care system in general and the cancer care community in particular to generate a change. It is time for the established medical community to look outside the conventional medicine box to explore the vast realm of integrative possibilities. It is also time for integrative oncology advocates—medical professionals and the general public—to become more intense in their advocacy.

A Request

This is an unusual request. Before you begin reading Chapter Three, I ask that you reread the analogy of the terrorist attacks at the opening of Chapter One. Review it with a new perspective. Compare every aspect of the story to the terror of cancer and our response to it. Contemplate it. Make your own analogies. Let it be a mental backdrop as you continue to read subsequent chapters. Reflect on the numbers. Memorize the basic statistics—cancers diagnosed, annually and daily as well as the number of cancer deaths, annually and daily. This will provide you with the basic perspective you need to effectively relate to the rest of this book. If you forget the numbers half way through the book, go back and review them.

Many of the statistics are conveniently listed in Appendix 3. We must all come to grips with the stark reality of this horrendous monster called cancer.

CHAPTER 3

THE CURRENT BATTLE
PLAN OF THE WAR

The conventional treatment for cancer has been surgery, chemotherapy, and radiation therapy for the last four or five generations of patients. Until just over a century ago, almost all cancers that were aggressively confronted involved some form of surgery. A tumor was removed and large areas around the affected tissue were cut away. In the early 1900s, the discovery of x-rays, radioactivity, and radium led to the use of radiation as a tumor fighter. Large areas of the body were bombarded with heavy one-time radiation that destroyed normal tissues as it attacked the tumors. The unbearable pain and morbid bodily disfigurement made the treatment much worse than the disease in many cases. In the 1920s, radiation administered in doses with improved equipment made its use more palatable and widespread. About mid-century, toxic chemicals injected into the body became a treatment of choice for many types of diseases including certain cancers. Again, primitive equipment and methodologies caused much harm to the patient from the debilitating drugs.

Looking backward from present day, we see the same basic approach to treating cancer. Certainly, physicians, researchers, and scientists have made notable discoveries and improvements in the methods and medicines used in this approach. But, relatively little exploration has been conducted beyond or outside of traditional conventional treatment.

Treatment Objectives

The decision of what treatment to choose is not always based on the potential to cure. Conventional treatments can be curative, adjuvant, or palliative.

Curative Treatment. The objective of curative treatment is to attempt to get rid of the cancer with the chosen treatment or mix of treatments. An example is removing a tumor completely by surgery and following up with chemotherapy to prevent recurrence.

Adjuvant Treatment. This treatment is used to enhance the effectiveness of a medication or other treatment. For instance, surgery may be used as an adjuvant treatment to reduce the size of a tumor in order to give chemotherapy a better chance of shrinking or eliminating it. Similarly, lasers may be used to activate a previously administered chemical that cancer cells have absorbed.

Palliative Treatment. A palliative treatment is often chosen if a cure is not thought possible. Any of a number of such treatments may be used to help the patient experience a higher quality of life. For example, radiation therapy and/ or chemotherapy may be prescribed to control cancer for a longer period of time, slowing the growth of tumors. Also, some surgeries can relieve the painful pressure of a tumor even though the tumor cannot be completely removed.

A common misconception of cancer treatment is that it all has the objective of ridding the body of the disease and attaining remission. In fact, much, if not most, treatment processes do not have curing as their goal. The mindset of most conventional treatment practitioners is that one of the three treatments above will be administered through one or more of the three methods below.

Surgery

As alluded to previously, cancer surgery has been with us for a few centuries. Perhaps the earliest historical highlight of its use was when Abigail Adams, daughter of the second president, John Adams, endured a grueling radical mastectomy in 1811 at the advice of the family physician. The operation was in the Adams' bedroom and was performed without anesthesia. It was virtually without precedence. She never recovered and died after three grueling years.

In the late 1800's, physicians began seriously exploring the potential of surgery as a typical solution for most cancer patients. Dr. William Halsted, known as the father of American surgery, began teaching and performing radical mastectomies for breast cancer in 1882. At that time, the consensus was that cancer masses grew and spread by producing "tentacles." These tentacles were thought to extend like tree roots into more of the affected organ or even to other parts of the body. Therefore, theoretically, if all tissue within the reach of the expanding tumor could be removed, the cancer could be eradicated. This concept was the basis for most cancer treatment well into the 20th century. From the turn of the century to the mid-1970's, about 90% of the women treated for breast cancer in the United States underwent a radical mastectomy (Wikipedia 2007).

Although early in the 20th century, researchers learned that cancer spread almost exclusively through the blood stream and lymphatic system, radical surgeries continued. The theory was that enough tissue should be removed beyond the affected area to ensure that no cancer cells were left to find their way into the blood vessels or lymphatic system. Any lymph ducts or lymph nodes near the tumor were often removed in case they might contain cancer cells from the tumor. Removal of part of the lymph system, however, had the negative effect of weakening the immune system.

The lymphatic system has a network of vessels and capillaries throughout the body that transports excess fluids, fat, and impurities from tissue cells to the blood circulatory system. The blood vessels then carry the potentially damaging materials to organs that eliminate them from the body. The lymphatic system, therefore, is a major component of the immune system. When any part of it is weakened or removed by surgery, it reduces the ability of the body to heal itself. So, the dilemma is whether it is more important to remove a possible carrier of cancer cells or retain a healthy immune system to fight the cells.

Over the last couple of decades, the trend in cancer surgery has been to do less radical surgery. Research has indicated that extraction of wide areas of tissue and large portions of the lymph system from an affected area is not usually necessary. Such extraction has been determined, in fact, to often be a detriment to healing. There seems to be more respect for the body's immune system as each year passes. However, numerous oncologists and surgeons continue to recommend radical surgery for malignant tumors. Conventional thinking in the medical world seems to be extremely difficult to change, regardless of the evidence. The syndrome tends to prevail that, if we have been doing it this way for years, it can't be wrong.

A Positive Treatment

Cancer surgery is sometimes the only treatment required, but more often is in conjunction with radiation and chemotherapy. Minor biopsy surgery removes all or part of a suspected tumor to determine whether it is malignant or benign. A surgeon may need to see the tumor and surrounding area to evaluate how advanced it is. Lymph nodes may have to be collected to determine whether the cancer cells have made their way into the lymph system. Even when a tumor has been well defined through technical means, but not qualified for complete removal, the doctor may need to remove as much as possible, a procedure called debulking. This debulking may prevent or slow life-threatening growth or it may make chemotherapy or radiation more effective. Palliative surgery, as stated before, may be to just improve quality of life—for example, to relieve pain from a tumor pressing a nerve, bone, or organ.

The most common cancer surgery is done as primary treatment. It is often considered the best chance for a cure, especially if it is localized within one organ. Where possible, the entire tumor is removed from the body along with surrounding tissue. Occasionally, a complete organ that is host to the cancer is removed. For instance, a lung lobe or complete lung may be removed if the body can continue to sustain itself with just the remaining lobes or the one lung. In the case of kidney cancer, a healthy second kidney would allow the taking of the other cancerous kidney. An option for prostate cancer is to remove the entire organ (prostatectomy), since it is not absolutely life sustaining.

If detected while the tumor is contained within a particular organ, surgery can often result in total remission. This is a best case scenario and would not require follow-on treatment. However, if there is potential that cancer cells have migrated to other parts of the body, chemotherapy and/or radiation will probably be recommended as a follow-on to the surgery.

Limitations

Of course, many categories of cancer are not tumor related, and, therefore, not candidates for surgery. Blood borne cancers, for instance, do not develop any masses or tissues that can be removed from the body by surgery.

Surgery is also not an option for many types of cancer tumors. Most cases of liver cancer cannot benefit from surgery due to essential blood vessels that cannot be disturbed. About 80% of all lung cancers are non-small-cell. The majority of non-small-cell lung cancers are inoperable. However, other techniques for removing tumors have been recently developed or are being researched. These include the use of liquid nitrogen to freeze the tumor (cryosurgery), and high-intensity laser light to vaporize cancer cells.

Harmful Side Effects

To better understand the risks that accompany cancer surgery, one needs to understand the fundamentals of tumor growth. All cells, malignant tumors included, must have a connection to the blood system. New tumors feed off the nearest capillaries carrying the blood. As the tumor matures, it develops its own blood vessels through a process called "angiogenesis." Angiogenesis is the process by which all tissues in the body grow new blood vessels for their survival. It is also instrumental in the healing of wounds, including surgery. Our regenerative ability to replace blood vessels and tissue are, of course, critical to our survival. This necessary process is our enemy, however, when it is helping tumors to survive. Receiving an ample supply of nutrients from new blood vessels, the tumor cells grow unnaturally and rapidly in comparison to healthy cells. Therefore, angiogenesis in the tumor area is a hindrance to fighting cancer.

A relatively recent medical discovery revealed that angiostatin and endostatin played a major role in combating tumors, especially those agitated by surgery.

Angiostatin is a natural protein in the body that inhibits the growth of blood vessels. It is also an important part of the blood clotting mechanism that keeps us from bleeding endlessly from a wound. Similarly, endostatin, also generated naturally by our bodies, works against angiogenesis and inhibits the growth of tumors. Therefore, both angiostatin and endostatin are natural tumor fighters. If a tumor does not have the ability to nourish itself, it cannot enlarge and indeed will shrink and eventually die. Surgery can often interfere with this natural attempt of the body to fight the cancerous tumor.

Removing a tumor significantly reduces the amount of angiostatin and endostatin available to the affected area. If any cancer cells remain in the area, or if some cells have metastasized beyond the area, angiostatin and endostatin that have their levels lowered from the surgery may not be sufficient to adequately attack blood vessel and tissue growth. Thus, the attempt of cancer surgery to rid the body of out-of-control tumors can have the opposing effect of also ridding the body of its natural healing properties. Clinical trials are being conducted at the time of this writing to determine if supplemental angiostatin, endostatin, or other anti-angiogenesis drug given before and/or after cancer surgery would prove beneficial. I will cover more on this subject in Chapter Six.

The pain that accompanies any surgery necessitates the use of analgesic pain drugs. This usually includes morphine, oxycodone, or other opiates. Such drugs impair the immune system and stimulate angiogenesis (new blood cell growth that feeds tumors). Unfortunately, these drugs are required at the time that optimal immune and anti-angiogenesis functions are critical to eradication of residual tumor cells that may have survived the surgery.

The same side effects that are experienced by patients of almost any surgery are often compounded with cancer surgery. Any time a major intrusion happens to the body, whether from surgery or injury, the immune system is preoccupied with that particular job and has less ability to counter other attacks. Fewer white blood cells and other components of the immune system are available to counter the cancer cells. Factor in the ever-increasing threat of staph infections, anesthesia complications, blood clots, blood transfusions, incision healing problems, and cancer surgery becomes a complex decision. Surgery is not for every cancer patient, and, for those qualified, it often fails to do the job.

Radiation

Shortly after the discoveries of radium, radioactivity, and x-rays, all within a few years of each other in the late 1800's, doctors began experimenting with the potential healing powers of radiation. The first cancer "cure" from radiation was reported in medical literature in 1899. This period is now viewed as the "Dark Ages" of radiation therapy evolution (Coosa Valley Technical College 2007). Doctors and medical technicians administered the therapy with little understanding of its dangerous effects. Large areas of patients' bodies were exposed to massive doses of radiation with hopes of destroying tumors in a single treatment. The process was debilitating, many deaths resulted, and tumor recurrence was high.

By the middle of the 20th Century, specific dosages had been identified and multiple treatments replaced the single treatment. The introduction of the vacuum x-ray tube led to the development of higher energy electrical devices that could deliver safer levels of radiation to deeper and better defined tissues and organs. Cobalt replaced radium as the radiation source. However, treatments continued to produce serious physical consequences such as severe skin damage, loss of energy, internal organ damage, and lack of appetite.

The computer boom and other technological advancements of the past few decades have vastly improved the safety and effectiveness of radiation therapy. Machines are now capable of delivering precise doses of radiation to tumors almost anywhere in the body with fewer side effects.

A Positive Treatment

Radiation therapy is most frequently used for the treatment of malignant tumors. It may also be targeted to lymph nodes if they are believed to contain cancer cells migrating from a tumor. Every attempt is made to radiate the tumor without damaging healthy tissues. Radiation beams are usually aimed from various angles toward the tumor in order to attack the tumor with larger doses than the surrounding and overlying tissue and organs receive.

The radiation damages the DNA of cells by ionizing, or de-energizing, the atoms which comprise the DNA. Cells normally repair damage on their own, but disrupting the DNA destroys or at least slows the cell's ability to repair itself. As long as the cells being radiated are tumor cells, radiation can be an effective weapon in the battle against the cancer.

There are three main types of radiation therapy: external beam radiotherapy, brachytherapy, and radioisotope therapy.

External beam radiotherapy is the most common and simplest method of delivery and has the longest history of use. It is the mainstay of radiation therapy. When most of us think of radiation therapy, we think of this method—an x-ray machine that sends beams of radiation into the body.

Brachytherapy is a more advanced cancer treatment where the radiation is sealed from surrounding healthy cells. Radioactive seeds are placed in or near the tumor itself, giving a high radiation dose to the tumor while reducing the radiation exposure in the surrounding healthy tissues. It is an especially advantageous technique for prostate, gynecologic, and head cancers where very critical tissues and organs are near the tumor.

Radioisotope therapy is unsealed, but is delivered through infusion into the bloodstream or ingested by mouth. It provides more protection to healthy cells than external beam, but less than brachytherapy. Radioisotope therapy is often chosen for cancers involving the thyroid and liver which interact closely with the blood system.

Some of the most celebrated advances in cancer treatment of recent years are in the domain of radiation therapy. Researchers have been concentrating on how best to selectively apply the radiation to the cancer cells without damaging healthy cells. They are progressing in the use of "radiolabeled" antibodies to deliver doses of radiation directly to the cancer site. Antibodies are proteins produced naturally by the body to combat antigens recognized by the immune system as foreign and undesired. The antibodies seek out the antigens and attack them. Some tumor cells contain these antigens that trigger the body's production of tumor-specific antibodies. Scientists are learning to attach radioactive substances to the antibodies in the laboratory and inject them into the cancer patient. The antibodies then transport the radioactive substances directly to the cancer cells where they can do their job without harming surrounding healthy cells.

Another potential radiation therapy breakthrough is hyperthermia. The use of heat in conjunction with radiation is being studied presently in university laboratories. Heat applied in tandem with radiation seems to increase the response rate of some tumors.

Limitations

The greatest limitation to radiation therapy is the collateral damage that is done to the healthy parts of the body. Even with brachytherapy and radioisotope therapy, some healthy cells will most likely be damaged.

Radiation therapy also causes a deficiency of oxygen in solid tumors. If the tumor is starved of oxygen, it will surge in its ability to repair itself. These oxygen deficient tumor cells become more capable of repairing the damage inflicted by the radiation. Therefore, the hypoxic tumor cells are more resistant to the effects of radiation.

Further frustrating researchers is the difficulty of identifying appropriate radioactive substances and determining safe and effective levels of radiation dosage. With every newly discovered process comes extensive experimentation to determine the parameters of application.

Harmful Side Effects

Although modern radiation therapy has as one of its primary objectives to minimize side effects, they continue to be an unfortunate downside of the treatment. The therapy, especially in higher doses, causes various side effects during treatment and for months or years after treatment.

During treatment, potentially severe damage may be done to the body's tissues including the skin, the throat, the guts, and the urinary tract. Typically the skin reddens and becomes sore a few days into the treatment. The skin may break down and become moist or oily. Temporary soreness and ulceration of the mouth and throat often occur. This can affect swallowing and require pain medication and nutritional support. Swelling of soft tissues is of particular concern during treatment of brain tumors which may already be pressing against the skull or brain. Temporary, and possibly permanent, infertility can result following direct exposure of ovaries or testicles to radiation.

Medium-term and long-term side effects include fibrosis from the scarring aspect of radiation. Hair loss, unlike that experienced from chemotherapy, is usually limited to the area treated. However, it is likely permanent. Wetness glands in the area of treatment will usually become dry. Salivary and tear glands dried up from head treatments severely reduce the patient's quality of life. Similarly, sweat glands in treated skin such as the armpit usually stop working. Naturally moist vaginal membranes often become dry following pelvic area radiation.

Radiation itself can be a cause of secondary malignancies in a small percentage of patients. It can weaken the immune system as it damages healthy cells, thereby making healthy cells vulnerable to becoming cancer cells.

Chemotherapy

In our context, chemotherapy is the use of cytotoxic drugs to treat cancer. Cytotoxic is the character of an agent that kills cells. A cytotoxic agent can be a chemical substance or natural immune cells. We all produce natural immune cells, or white blood cells, which constantly seek out infectious or other harmful cells in our bodies and destroy them. That is how we stay well or get well when we are sick. These same natural cells in our blood system attack cancer cells. Cytotoxic drugs infused into the body also have the objective of killing cancer cells. Unfortunately, they also kill healthy cells, including immune cells, in the process. The chemotherapy concept is that cytotoxic drugs can kill enough of the cancer cells to justify the damage to other cells.

The first drug used for chemotherapy was not originally intended for that purpose. Mustard gas was used extensively on the battle fields of Europe during World War I. During further experiments with the chemical as a potential weapon in World War II, some people were accidentally exposed to it and studied to determine its effect. They were found to have a very low white blood cell count. Researchers believed that the chemical might have the same destructive effect on cancer cells. Several patients with advanced lymphomas (blood-borne cancers) were injected with the chemical and made remarkable, although temporary, improvement. Shortly, other drugs were tested to treat cancer. Drug development since then has become a multi-billion-dollar industry. Chemotherapy has revolutionized cancer treatment. But, many of the limitations of its use that plagued its early development still apply.

A Positive Treatment

Generally, most chemotherapy drugs work by impairing cell division. They target rapidly dividing cells. Some drugs cause cancer cells to undergo "apoptosis" or cell suicide. Combined modality chemotherapy is used with other cancer treatments such as surgery or radiation therapy. Combination chemotherapy treats patients with several different drugs simultaneously through differing mechanisms and with varying side effects. This minimizes the potential of resistance of cancer cells to any one agent.

Initial chemotherapy is usually aimed at shrinking or eliminating the primary tumor. Subsequent regimens may be employed to counter any spread that might have occurred in other parts of the body. Since spreading, or metastasizing, tumors are usually in their rapidly-dividing stage, they are more susceptible to chemical attack. Palliative chemotherapy is often prescribed for patients diagnosed with terminal cancer. It is given without curative intent, but rather to decrease the tumors and increase life expectancy.

Determining the type and dose of chemical to use is an extremely complex process. The molecular make up of the tumor or cancer cells calls for different chemical mixes. Certain chemicals are best for certain levels of cancer cell or tumor development. The physical and emotional strength of the patient will dictate the toleration levels of certain chemicals. A particular category of chemicals is selected for attempts to eliminate the cancer, while another category is required to combat cancer spread, and yet another category exists for palliative care.

Delivery of chemotherapy is most often intravenous, although many agents can be administered orally. In some cases, isolated delivery through direct injection is accomplished. As in brachytherapy, this is frequently done for treatment of liver or lung cancers where high doses are needed while avoiding collateral damage to surrounding tissues. Depending on the patient, the type and stage of cancer, and the type and dosage of chemicals, chemotherapy may be performed on either an inpatient or outpatient basis.

Constant, large-scale efforts are on-going to find chemical combinations targeted at specific types of cancer. Clinical trials at major cancer centers are resulting in both the extension and quality of life among cancer patients. These trials pursue more effective, less toxic solutions to cancer treatment. They also disprove the efficacy of treatments that do not pass the scrutiny of the research.

Limitations

The principal dilemma of chemotherapy practitioners and patients is how to attack the tumor without harming the rest of the body. Numerous complementary therapy options are available that work in harmony with chemotherapy while reducing its negative effects. Hyperthermia can increase its effectiveness, hypnotherapy and acupuncture can reduce its some of its side effects, and nutrients can boost the immune system to lessen the duration of treatment, just to highlight a few. However, lack of universal acceptance of many such practices and the substantial research that is still needed in their integration limits their use. Until integrative therapy becomes the credible treatment of choice by doctors and patients alike, the solution to cancer will continue to escape us.

Another challenge for chemotherapy providers is selecting the correct balance of drug options. Factors including physical and emotional health of the patient, type and maturity of the cancer, and reaction to the side effects all contribute to the complexity of determining the drug mix.

A third limitation is the difficulty of aligning the type of chemical with the type of tumor or cancer cell. Some tumors or cancer cells are highly resistant to particular chemotherapy drugs. Yet, unless a drug has been specifically proven to be effective against a particular type of cancer, often a less effective drug is chosen as a default solution.

Harmful Side Effects

The best way I know to describe the debilitating nature of chemotherapy is to reference my personal experiences. The following is a brief account of the three years my former wife suffered under the oppression of aggressive chemotherapy.

Although I have not been personally subjected to the procedure, I lived it day and night, week after week, month after month with my then best friend and soul mate.

Immediately after receiving the first infusion, Connie became nauseated. Even when nausea can be controlled to an extent, it usually takes days or weeks before the dosage and anti-nausea supplements can be adjusted to individual tolerance and need. The vomiting and diarrhea were devastating for the first several treatments. She was confined to the bed for days. Hardly anything she ate would stay with her. Her oncologist worked vigorously at customizing the chemicals and the nausea medicine to balance her needs and tolerance levels. Even after finding the best combination of dosages, she continued to have occasional regressive bouts with nausea.

When the nausea was in check, lack of appetite still plagued the pursuit of healthy nutrition. Connie had to force herself to eat without any feeling of hunger. The food she was able to eat was virtually tasteless. Enjoying a meal and favorite snack treats are some of life's simplest pleasures that we often take for granted. Imagine weeks and months looking on any food item with disgust. I had to be covert in even preparing myself a sandwich, because the smell of food from another room would cause her to gag or vomit. Her appetite gradually improved somewhat with her body's reluctant acceptance of the therapy. But, meals were never a pleasurable experience as long as chemicals were being infused. After several treatments, mouth sores, a common side effect of chemotherapy, made eating a painful experience and provided further incentive to not take in enough food.

Fatigue was another major challenge. Connie had been an athletic person with seemingly boundless energy. Throughout the chemo regimen, she was constantly tired. After the lightest task, she would have to lie down on the couch or recline in a chair for a while before attempting anything else. Early bedtimes and late risings were strange new characteristics of her sleep habits. Social activities virtually ceased, since a few minutes of standing and small talk would exhaust her. Mental depression was not the culprit in any of these symptoms. Although she had every reason and right to be depressed, Connie was amazingly upbeat and thinking positively during her battle. She was just physically drained from the chemical attack on her body.

From the beginning of treatment, a weak immune system caused by a low white blood cell count often kept her from being near other people. As the level of impact of some of the other side effects became more tolerable, the cumulative effect of the chemo began to more severely restrict the immune system. The oncologist directed bi-weekly white cell counts. The white blood cells are made in the bone marrow and circulate in the bloodstream to attack bad bacteria and other undesirables in the body. Generally, chemotherapy kills many types of healthy and important cells indiscriminately as it attempts to kill cancer cells. It usually interferes with the bone marrow's production of white blood cells. Since the white cells are essential to the body's immune system, a chemotherapy patient is typically much more vulnerable to infections. If a patient develops an infection, chemo treatments are usually ceased until the infection is under control. If this happens, the cancer gets a reprieve to re-energize and grow. Connie went through these cycles several times. A normal white blood cell count is 4,000 to

11,000. Hers was often measured in the low hundreds. When they were in those low numbers, she would be restricted to the house by doctor's orders unable to personally interface with anyone except me for fear of infection.

The white blood cell damage is one of the principal things that make chemotherapy such a "catch-22." It is supposedly the answer, but is also the problem. Cancer, like most other undesirable abnormalities in our bodies must be counter attacked by the strongest immune system that we can muster against it. A robust immune system is imperative in controlling the chaotic growth of cancer cells. Just when we need our immune system to be at its peak to fight errant cancer cells, we effectively shut it down with chemicals. Now the debate remains whether the ultimate good of chemical intervention which kills good and bad cells outweighs the ultimate good of a healthy immune system, perhaps enhanced by natural supplements. Most doctors will say it does; naturopaths will say it does not. This debate is probably endless.

The Cumulative Effect

I could not possibly relate all of the pros and cons of conventional cancer treatment in a chapter. My personal experience with Connie's treatment could fill another book. I conclude this chapter with some final comments on the combined treatment she encountered.

The treatment and its impact on our lives were the worst experiences I had faced in my life at that point. Today, I can assure that its devastating effect was eclipsed only by Connie's death. And, of course, my experience was nothing compared to what she had to deal with. I must, however, touch on the psycho-social aspect of what we went through during our three-year battle.

Before Connie was diagnosed, we had been partners in a military career spanning 24 years. A huge part of the role of a career officer involved relationship building through social events and activities. After retiring from the Air Force, I became a pastor on the staff of a large church in our community. There, our responsibility for building relationships was perhaps even more critical than in the military. So, throughout our adult lives, we had been immersed in constant interface with other people. We were a gregarious couple by nature and by necessity. We craved fellowship with friends and acquaintances and found fulfillment in it. Suddenly, the words, "you have cancer," turned our whole lifestyle upside-down. Initially, the frequent consultations and treatments took our priorities away from the lives of others— our friends, even our family. Later the sickness, the pain, and the confinement kept us isolated to a great degree. Of course, there were phone calls, cards, and letters, but face-to-face encounters were greatly diminished. For anyone, especially those who love to be around people, conventional cancer treatment is usually accompanied by feelings of alienation, disconnection, loneliness, and even guilt. Physical distress coupled with psycho-social grief is a poor foundation from which to build a healing force to combat cancer.

Collateral damage to the body is another serious concern of traditional, conventional cancer treatment. Many medical procedures are accompanied by risks of injury to otherwise healthy parts of the body. For any chemo treatment of more than a few days or weeks, oncologists usually recommend that a "port" be installed through which to inject the chemical mixture. Repeated intravenous infusion of chemicals and drawing of blood directly into and from vessels at various locations become impractical after several days. A port is a small, round disc made of plastic or metal that is placed under your skin. A catheter connects the port to a large vein, most often in the chest. The caregiver inserts a needle into the port to give the chemotherapy or to draw blood. This port installation procedure is usually accomplished without incident. However, it does require the surgeon to operate very near the lungs. In Connie's case, the highly qualified surgeon punctured her lung in the process of port insertion. This is a rare occurrence, but just one of several anomalies that can violate the body during conventional treatment. There are few injuries more painful than a punctured lung, and the remedy is even more painful. The lung has to heal itself over a period of a week to ten days while an aspirator hose inserted through the diaphragm continuously drains fluid. The patient never gets out of bed and can hardly move during the process. Of course, all chemotherapy is halted during the repair, again giving the cancer time to recharge.

Yet, another ever-looming threat of collateral misfortune is that of serious, even deadly, infection. Any surgery runs the risk of infection, especially when the immune system is already weakened by other treatments. Additionally, infection around the port is something doctors have to watch for constantly. The actual condition that caused the precipitous slide that ended Connie's life was a bacterial infection so potent that the strongest antibiotics could not faze it. Doctors surmised that the infection was contracted through some part of the invasive cancer treatment. She developed a septic condition that laid siege to her entire body. The full month of antibiotic experimentation to try to eliminate the infection allowed the cancer to grow unconstrained. Even though the official cause of her death was metastasis of breast cancer, it was an infection, probably from the treatment, that led to the ultimate loss of the battle.

There are numerous collateral effects of cancer treatment that exacerbate the already traumatic experiences associated with the disease. The three that we encountered just added yet more heartaches to our world ravaged by cancer at that time.

Without question, tremendous progress has been made in the three compartments of conventional cancer treatment. The disease would have probably eliminated almost every victim whose life it invaded had they not had the physicians and scientists who have dedicated their lives to this sector of medicine. The question is whether this conventional treatment alone is our best shot in the fight. Are we as a nation doing the best we can as fast as we can in this war. Are we on track to really defeat cancer or are we just keeping up with it? Is it still a draw? Are we in a quagmire?

CHAPTER 4

THE QUAGMIRE OF THE WAR

The cost of wars in money and lives is always an issue for any nation, especially one as democratic as the United States. As the American people became weary and frustrated with the Vietnam War, opponents began referring to it as a "quagmire." The prolonged fighting and spending didn't seem to be bringing us closer to victory or even a hope of victory. Literally, a quagmire is ground that is mushy causing anyone attempting to pass over it to sink into it. It renders the person almost unable to move if not completely stuck. Figuratively, it is a very annoying and disturbing situation that drastically slows or stops progress. Those who oppose the wars in Iraq and Afghanistan frequently refer to them as "another Vietnam-like quagmire."

People slogging in a quagmire make a valiant effort to continue moving forward, but the harder they try, the less progress they seem to make. At best, the meager results do not justify the vast amount of energy applied to the effort. Continuing to plod through the mess, the travelers will not likely see what could be solid ground to the side or low branches overhead that could be used to rescue them from their desperate situation. They are totally focused on where they are rather than on what might be within reach.

I believe the quagmire that has characterized wars against our nation's enemies also applies to the war on cancer. What seemed promising decades ago has not materialized as the ultimate solution, yet the medical community continues, in many ways, to pursue the course with limited results.

People's frustrations with the slow progress are increasingly showing up in the media. A 2008 cover story in *U.S. News and World Report* magazine entitled, "Breaking Cancer's Code," presented a rather positive angle on the latest research. A reader who had lost her husband to cancer leaving her to raise their two small children alone wrote in a response letter to the editor:

> I'm tired of reading of the rah-rah tone of coverage of the progress in cancer treatment. Cancer still kills a lot of people who remain anonymous amid the cheerleading.

A 2009 article in *The New York Times*, "Advances Elusive in the Drive to Cure Cancer," gave a pessimistic view of the war:

> Cancer has always been an expensive priority. Since the war on cancer began, the National Cancer Institute, the federal government's main cancer research entity, with 4,000 employees, has alone spent $105 billion. And other government agencies, universities, drug companies, and philanthropies have chipped in uncounted billions more. Yet the death rate for cancer, adjusted for the size and age of the population, dropped only 5 percent from 1950 to 2005. In contrast, the death rate for heart disease dropped 64 percent in that time, and for flu and pneumonia, it fell 58 percent. Still the perception, fed by the medical profession and its marketers, and by popular sentiment, is that cancer can almost always be prevented. If that fails, it can usually be treated, even beaten.

Historical Responses to Cancer

To rescue ourselves from a quagmire, we must understand what got us to that point, then try to determine why we are still there. The longer the tradition of any activity, the harder it is to change. When people become comfortably familiar with something over a long period of time, they are naturally resistant, or at least apathetic, toward much of anything different. The tendency is to follow the tradition and tune out any suggestions of other options. The status quo is usually the easiest course, but seldom the best.

Winner of the MacArthur Prize for public health, author, and leading cancer authority Michael Lerner, in his book *Choices in Healing*, makes the following observation:

More often than not, cancer patients believe that their choices for therapy are dictated by the findings of pure biomedical science. Cancer patients also tend to believe that biomedical science is a monolith—a huge body of knowledge that dictates what an individual must do with a specific kind of cancer—and that all the information generated by this monolithic science is funneled into the brains of the first physicians they consult. Neither belief is accurate.

I endorse Lerner's conclusion from personal experience:

This perfectly describes Connie and me at the time she was first diagnosed with breast cancer. We assumed that the rather narrow application of conventional treatment prescribed by our oncologist was the only option. In fact, this assumption drove our approach to her treatment for almost three years. Until just prior to her death, we continued to believe that conventional medicine alone was the only choice we had. There was never any advice offered concerning CAM or integrative options. We were not advised about diet, immune system enhancement, supplemental vitamins and herbs, acupuncture, clinical trial participation, vaccines, hormonal therapy, coping with stress, pain management, etc. Furthermore, we were naively unaware that the clinical regimen we were undergoing had changed very little in the past half-century. We had been prescribed the traditional standard treatment of surgery, radiation, and chemotherapy, and we never considered that there could be other therapy options or complements.

The International Perspective

Other advanced nations appear to be making their way out of this quagmire of traditional cancer treatment. Is there a clue to be found in the quest for the solution to cancer by looking beyond our borders? Even within conventional treatment, is our strategy sound compared to that of other nations?

A look at the differences in cancer therapies practiced among leading industrial nations clearly establishes the United States medical community as the most aggressive. But aggressiveness is not always a good thing, especially in conventional cancer treatment. Most major European countries maintain a medical culture of less interference in the aesthetics and functions of the body. European doctors will almost always opt for a gentler approach to everything from colds to catastrophic diseases.

Lynn Payer, author of *Medicine and Culture*, compares and contrasts the practice of medicine in the U.S. and Europe. In his foreword to Payer's book, Dr. Kerr White, a physician and leading researcher for Health Services Research wrote that "only about 15% of all contemporary medical interventions are supported by objective clinical evidence that they do more good than harm." Most medical practices are reflections of culture—culture of the physicians and culture of the patients.

The thrust of Payer's *Medicine & Culture* is to demonstrate how the U.S. and three other industrial countries; England, France, and Germany; differ in their practice of medicine, particularly in the treatment of cancer. The differences are because of their national culture, history, and medical training.

In her introduction, Payer refers to a survey where British and American oncologists were asked how they personally would want to be treated if they had various cancers. For advanced bladder cancer, 92% of American doctors wanted radical surgery compared to only 30% of British doctors. In the case of prostate cancer, 79% of American doctors and 4% of British doctors would opt for radical surgery (Payer 1988). This says volumes about the way cancer is treated in the two countries and the way their respective oncologists have been educated.

Payer observed that the French place a high priority on the health of the body and its ability to fight disease. She writes, "[this belief] also undoubtedly plays a role in the fact that fewer invasive procedures are used in intensive care units in France than in the United States—with patients doing equally well in both countries." (Harris Interactive 2007)

German physicians consider poor circulation to be the underlying cause of many diseases of specific organs. Hydrotherapy—hot and cold whirlpool baths—are prescribed to remedy blood pressure problems and, therefore, many internal diseases. According to Payer, "Still another legacy of romanticism to Germany medicine is the healing powers accorded to nature, whether it be in the form of long walks in the forests, mud baths, or herbal medicine." (Harris Interactive 2007)

Payer noted the aggressive, "if in doubt, do a lot" philosophy of the United States' medical culture:

> The aggressive approach that has characterized American medicine was evident even before the American Revolution. Dr. Benjamin Rush (a friend of Presidents Jefferson and Adams) believed that one of the hindrances to the development of medicine had been an "undue reliance upon the powers of nature in curing disease." Rush's success in promulgating his thesis meant that for many years to come, massive purging and bloodletting were to characterize American medical practice (Harris Interactive 2007).

By the way, Dr. Benjamin Rush was the doctor who recommended the radical mastectomy of Abigail Adams referenced in Chapter Three. In a letter to Abigail's parents, he wrote, "Let there be no delay in flying to the knife."

Payer quotes a British medical student training in a modern American hospital:

> There seemed to be an overwhelming number of so-called 'type A' personalities around—and the only explanation I could offer for this was that American medicine selects, and is selected by, a different type

of student than in England. ….American medicine is aggressive partly because doctors are trained to be aggressive but also because many patients equate aggressive with better (Harris Interactive 2007).

The medical playing field seems to be leveling somewhat between the United States and other industrial nations since Lynn Payer conducted her research in the 1990s. As cancer specialists from other countries acknowledge that their cancer survival rates continue to lag behind those of the United States, their trends are shifting to a more aggressive approach to treatment. The latest reports suggest that cancer care in Europe is improving and that the gaps between countries are narrowing. However, the United States survival rates in general are still higher than those of any country in Europe.

An analysis led by Dr. Arduino Verdecchia of the National Center for Epidemiology, Health Surveillance, and Promotion, in Rome, Italy, involved almost seven million patients from 21 European countries diagnosed with cancer between 2000 and 2002. The age-adjusted 5-year survival rates were 47% for men and 56% for women. This is considerably lower than the United States Surveillance, Epidemiology, and End Results (SEER) analysis rates of 66% for men and 63% for women. Dr. Verdecchia commented that that analysis also showed that the wide variations across countries, which have persisted for many years, "might be on the verge of decreasing." (Medscape Medical News 2007). This would seem to affirm the more aggressive treatment concept in America, but, let's look further.

A logical conclusion might be that the more aggressive treatment in the U.S. is responsible for the greater survivability. Looking further into the gap in survival rates between other countries and the U.S., and the trend toward other countries in closing that gap, the conclusions are not necessarily obvious. In reality, almost all of the variations in survival rates and the narrowing of the gaps have little to do with the levels of aggressiveness in treatment. The statistics have everything to do with prevention and early detection. *Lancet Oncology*, a respected world-wide monthly medical journal, reported that the Italian study's disparity in survival rates was largely due to "differences in the timeliness of diagnosis." (Medscape Medical News 2007) Much more intensive screening for cancer in the United States (mammograms, colonoscopies, and PSA tests) and the resultant early treatment account for virtually all of the survivability advantage in the U.S. Dr. Verdecchia and his colleagues concluded that the causes of the differences in rates were organization, training, professional skills, application of evidence-based guidelines, investment in diagnostic and treatment facilities and tumor stage (Medscape Medical News 2007). Notice that the differences are assumed to have little or nothing to do with treatment methodology, chemicals used, radiation, or surgery.

It seems that the U.S. has made impressive strides in getting patients to discover their cancer earlier and in developing a more sophisticated infrastructure. Both of these improvements have brought us slightly higher survivability rates compared to other industrialized nations. But, whether the national culture of the medical community is overly aggressive or cautiously conservative appears to matter little in the survival of cancer patients. I suggest that, if everything but the treatment protocol were factored out of the data, the survival rates would be virtually equal internationally. Some countries would rely more than others on CAM practices and other countries would rely more on chemicals, radiation, and surgery. All would be equally successful.

If I were destined to have cancer, would I want to be in the United States? Absolutely! But, only because I would probably know about it sooner and be able to treat it as I chose before it advanced. That is the advantage of being a cancer patient in this country. The disadvantage is dealing with the narrow mindset of limited treatment options, most of which are devastating to the body, mind, and spirit.

A Strategy Shift Is Always Difficult

There is an interesting similarity between the relatively recent transition in the conduct of military operations and the transition needed in the war against cancer. Until early in the 20th Century, the strategy of military leaders for thousands of years was largely to overwhelm the enemy with waves of combatants and powerful weaponry. The goal was to shock and intimidate. There have been attempts throughout history to promote alternatives to such an aggressive strategy. The Bible's Old Testament records a few examples of the Israelites using surprise, flanking movements, dispersing of troops, attacking from the rear, etc. to win their battles. The Chinese sixth century BC war strategist, Sun Tsu, wrote about being creative in battle and bringing the unexpected to the enemy. Still, through the ages, by far the most common war strategy and battle tactic involved two armies in frontal assault combat bringing all their might against each other until one was defeated. Machiavelli, the Italian philosopher and strategist of the 16th century endorsed this ruthless, brute force strategy described as the only way to prevail over evil societies and nations. We see this in paintings and movie re-enactments of medieval fighting, the Revolutionary War, and the Civil War. Men charge at each other in mass, then collide wielding swords or discharging weapons at close range in bloody, high casualty combat.

A significant change in strategy and tactics took place in World War 1. With the invention of the machine gun, artillery, and tank, close range musket and bayonet fighting along with the principle of mass had to be rethought. Forces became more spread out over the battle field. Fox holes and trenches were dug for cover. The coordinated mix of ground troops, tanks, and airplanes during World War II formed a new paradigm of war strategy. Certainly, the conventional strategy of overwhelming power continued to dominate both world wars. But later in Korea and Vietnam, and especially in Iraq and Afghanistan, special forces using covert methods became very important to the commanders. As the opposition changes, so must the defense tactics. With terrorism as our main present day threat, we now face an elusive enemy with no geographical limitation, no ethical restraint, and no observable strategy. Today's terrorists certainly don't fight with heavy weapons at known positions. Substantial conventional warfare capability is still rightly maintained, but we are now developing more flexible, lower cost unconventional forces targeted specifically to the threat.

Heavy tanks and field artillery continue to have utility, but flexible troops with protective light weight vests and night vision optics are becoming the priority for the new battlefield. The roles of manned supersonic fighter jets and strategic bombers are being complemented by small unmanned aerial vehicles (UAVs) controlled from the ground. Lighter, swifter, cheaper, and more adaptable combat forces are the strategic components of choice for the enemy we face today. These forces have the ability to strike surgically with minimal collateral damage while incurring much lower levels of risk. Without completely abandoning the capability for the "shock and awe" necessary for the first days of the Iraq war, our defense research and funding are wisely being increased in the "seek and destroy" capability of unconventional systems.

Likewise, conventional cancer treatment has been the mainstay of the medical community since the earliest theories of how to combat the disease. However, since the 1950's entrepreneurial practitioners in the field have studied and applied myriad options other than, or in addition to, conventional methods for the treatment. Even though many of these complementary or alternative methods have shown real promise, few have been taken seriously. Even fewer have been researched and tested in credible scientific labs. Like the military establishment's initial response to unconventional warfare, the conventional medical establishment has for years labeled most integration of complementary methods as unworthy of attention or even quackery. Not until recently have complements to conventional treatment been considered a serious subject of debate. Genuine progress in medicine, particularly cancer treatment, is being restrained by old thinking about new strategies. The established practitioners generally stand in staunch defense of their methodologies.

The Public Spin

As a former military officer who is still a close observer of military operations, I understand and appreciate that, from the Secretary of Defense to the basic recruit, there is a need to put the best face on a war. As battle losses amass, the public affairs spin emphasizes the progress that is being made and the enemy death toll. Although our own setbacks may be matters of record, the leadership hierarchy purposely avoids stating the obvious, choosing to instead focus on the incremental advances that are taking place. Astute reporters discern such bias. As a previously referenced article in *The New York Times* noted, "Still, the perception, fed by the medical profession and its marketers, and by popular sentiment, is that cancer can almost always be prevented. If that fails, it can usually be treated, even beaten."

Similarly, the major institutions and organizations of the medical community regularly make celebrative announcements about new positive cancer findings and statistics that are echoed by local offices. They ensure that the media herald any news of decreases in mortality rates from the latest data. But, the most observant citizens see through the news releases and recognize the relativity and reality of the information.

A major announcement from the principal annual report on cancer trends recently swept through the wires and airways of journalism. Since it takes over three years for the data to be organized, analyzed, and presented, new news is actually old news when reporting on medical statistics. This *Annual Report to the Nation on the Status of Cancer, 1975-2005* was released in December, 2008. It was the yearly collaborative effort of the NCI, the ACS, The Centers for Disease Control and Prevention, and the North American Association of Central Cancer Registries. The news release stated:

> For the first time since the report was first issued in 1998, both incidence and death rates for all cancers combined are decreasing for both men and women.

The report continued:

> Although cancer death rates have been dropping since the publication of the first Annual Report to the Nation ten years ago, the latest edition marks the first time the report has documented a simultaneous decline in cancer incidence, the rate at which new cancers are diagnosed, for both men and women. Based on the long-term incidence trend, rates for all cancers combined decreased 0.8 percent per year from 1999 through 2005.... Death rates from cancer fell an average of 1.8 percent each year from 2002 to 2005 according to the new report (ACS Advisory 2008).

The New York Times headline for covering this report read, "Lengthy Fall in U.S. Cancer Rates a First." John Niederhuber, director of the NCI was quoted in the article, "We're moving in the right direction....This is not just a blip on the screen." (Rabin 2008)

Now, I want to be counted among the first to applaud decreases in both the cancer incidence and death rates. I pray that they both decrease significantly every year. This news was far better than increasing rates or even a rate plateau. However, after appropriate celebration and credit where credit is due, let's put it in perspective that gives us plenty of reason to fight even harder.

The details of the report credit most of the historic 0.8 percent diagnosis rate decrease to promotion efforts toward healthier lifestyles, screening, and early detection. We seem to be doing better in those areas. Everywhere we turn, we see and hear admonitions to eat healthier, exercise more, avoid tobacco, get regular mammograms and colorectal screenings, and avoid known carcinogens. Experts were also quick to caution that this decrease in incidence rate may to some degree reflect inconsistent screening practices causing some cancers that used to be detected to now go undiagnosed. The strategic director for cancer surveillance at the ACS, Ahmedin Jemal, went so far as to say, "This might not be good news. It's always difficult to interpret the incidence rate."

The decreased mortality rate should also be looked at in perspective. A 1.8 percent annual decrease in the number of cancer deaths means that, of the over 1500 cancer deaths each day, 27 fewer are dying today than on a typical day last year. If one of us were among those 27, we would, of course, be rejoicing. Nevertheless, we are still losing over 1500 Americans each day to the disease.

That 1.8 percent becomes even less impressive as we consider another statistic. It turns out that most of that 1.8 percent overall decrease was linked to a few of the most common cancers—prostate at 4.4 percent, colon/rectum at 2.6 percent, breast at 2.1 percent, and lung at 2.0 percent. The report attributed much of these particular decreases to the changes in risk factors and screening patterns. Non-treatment advances highlighted as contributing to the better survival rates were (1) a pronounced fall in number of smokers,

(2) greater participation in mammograms, (3) more Pap tests, (4) alternatives to postmenopausal hormone therapy, and (5) pursuit of more active lifestyles. There was only one mention of gains in new treatments as being factors in the better survivability rate (NCI 2008).

So, again, the fact that a few more people are surviving cancer has little to do with treatment breakthroughs and everything to do with earlier diagnosis and a healthier lifestyle. When exercise, better nutrition, and ending bad habits prevent the occurrence of cancer, it is like diplomacy easing pressure on the battlefield. It helps, but it is not bringing victory. When screening and testing detect cancer at an early stage, it is like military intelligence discovering enemy plans and thwarting them before they can cause great harm. For the most part, positive news in the war against cancer is from aggressive efforts in diplomacy and intelligence. We are preventing it better and finding it earlier. Unfortunately, the 1.4 million Americans who are being diagnosed with cancer each year have not been able to prevent it. Most of them don't catch it in the early stages and, therefore, have to subject themselves to very aggressive treatment. Almost half of them suffer through lengthy and debilitating efforts to beat the disease only to experience defeat and die. Each year in this country our casualties from cancer continue to outnumber our casualties from World War I and World War II combined. And, we press on with the same tired, 50-year-old strategy.

Of course, we all commend the successes in preventing thousands of potential cancer battles from happening. Perhaps I and many reading this book would be making regular visits to treatment centers right now if we lived in the health environment of a few years ago. And similarly, I acknowledge the great strides made in early detection which have allowed thousands to defeat their cancer before it had the opportunity to organize and fully deploy its formidable forces. But, the war still rages. Well over a half million cancer patients each year fight ugly, drawn out battles just to eventually pay the ultimate cost exacted by the disease—death.

We keep fighting and fighting and fighting a war that drains our nation's human and financial resources. The diplomacy of prevention and the intelligence of early detection are easing the casualty count somewhat at the periphery.

But, real victory hangs on defeating the enemy through treatment—killing the evil cells and enhancing the body's ability to fight. It is here that the same old conventional warfare strategy that we have used for a half century has failed us. Its positives are far outweighed by its negatives. We are in a quagmire in the war against cancer. We are slipping, spinning around, and bogging down. Yet, many call it progress and ask for more support to pursue the same strategy. It is time for a strategy change. It is time to develop and deploy the unconventional special forces to fight both separately from and along side of conventional forces. Let's now take an honest look at this new strategy in the next chapters.

PART 2

THE NEW STRATEGY OBJECTIVES

CHAPTER 5

THE PRACTICE OF
NUTRITIONAL TACTICS

P art Two will transition us from the stalemate status of cancer treatment to the potential solutions for that stalemate. The new and promising approach to cancer treatment must involve CAM therapies administered as integrative treatment by trained and experienced oncologists. Later, I will review organized opposition that CAM and integrative treatment has been up against over the years. But first, it is important that you become familiar with the types of complementary protocols that are either available or developing. These are examples critical to the new strategy for the war on cancer.

Diet and Nutrition

It is universally understood and accepted that even young, disease-free bodies must have a balanced, nutritious diet to grow strong and remain healthy. As will be discussed later, cancer treatment patients usually experience nausea, loss of appetite, and various eating interferences. This frequently leads to malnutrition which is often harder on the body than the cancer. If a healthy body requires ample nutrition, and a cancerous body has greater need, but less desire for it, ensuring optimum nutrition for cancer patients is critical. Yet, nutrition seldom receives high priority in conventional cancer treatment.

Probably the most commonly referenced and least controversial complementary or integrative approach to cancer treatment is to eat the right foods. Still, many oncologists remain skeptical about the efficacy of a particular diet in relation to treatment. However, it is accepted within most conventional medical circles that a diet rich in phytonutrients, isothiocyanates, dietary fiber, and Omega-3 fatty acids is important in <u>preventing</u> cancer. You may not be familiar with the first two big words.

Phytonutrients include antioxidants, anticarcinogens, and bioflavonoids. These properties are found in the general categories of fruits, green leafy vegetables, beans, and whole grains. Soy beans contain phytonutrients that may protect against hormone sensitive cancers by blocking receptors with plant estrogens and other inhibitors naturally present in the beans. Isothiocyanates have similar properties that are found in broccoli, cabbage, cauliflower, and kale. Dietary fiber is the indigestible part of plant foods found in whole grain cereals, breads, nuts, and seeds. It is not only good for colon health, but also dilutes dangerous carcinogenic substances and invites "friendly" bacteria. Omega-3 fatty acids in oily fish such as salmon, halibut, and tuna are proven to be a health protector. Regular intake of foods with these qualities is recommended by virtually all researchers for protection against the onset of cancer. Whether such foods are effective in treatment is more controversial.

Since the medical community is almost unanimous in its agreement that a nutritious diet of low fat, high fiber whole foods with fresh vegetables and fruits reduces the risk of most cancers, isn't it worth exploring the effect of such a diet on existing cancers? Should a moderate diet, rich in anti-cancer nutrients that health professionals recommend to prevent cancer, not be considered for a more aggressive, therapeutic program for those that already have cancer? Yet, controlled, clinical trials of radical therapeutic diets receive a cool reception in mainstream medicine.

Richard Nahin of the National Center for Complementary and Alternative Medicine (NCCAM) was one of the authors of the 2007 CDC alternative medicine study referenced in Chapter 2. He described the study's findings of increased use of alternative remedies as "pretty amazing." Then, he cautioned,

"However, it is difficult to say if the level of use is harmful or beneficial because many therapies have not undergone rigorous scientific testing to gauge their effectiveness." (Stobbe 2008) One of the most common mantras of the medical science community is that people are moving away from traditional medicine, but we don't know whether that is good or bad, since very little outside of traditional medicine is being adequately tested.

The NCI estimates that 35% or more of all cancers have a nutritional connection (Cancer Nutrition Center 2007). Furthermore, the NCI says an astounding 20% to 40% of cancer patients die from causes related to malnutrition, not from the cancer itself, and 80% have some form of clinical malnutrition. Unfortunately, too frequently, conventional medical advice suggests that patients eat whatever they want without much regard to nutrition. Acting on this advice can actually feed the patient's cancer, promote their malnutrition, and contribute to the patient's inability to tolerate treatment. If the malnutrition is not addressed, it can cause "cachexia," a syndrome that compromises immunity, produces weakness, and causes loss of weight, fat, and muscle (PR Web 2008).

I had this experience:

My head was filled from researching naturopathic sources on the internet and at the library. Our oncologist had mentioned nothing about diet during treatment. I finally caught her in the hallway with a spare moment and ask her what my wife, Connie, should be eating during her chemo treatments. She said it was most important for patients to eat whatever they wanted and could tolerate because chemotherapy suppresses the patient's appetite. I told her that I had read that sugar and white flour foods should be avoided by cancer patients. She remained adamant that we should not be concerned about diet as that was the least of our worries during cancer treatment. She was right that cancer patients need nourishment, because the treatment itself leads to malnutrition. But to conclude that, therefore, the patient should eat anything and everything is, as I have learned since, completely wrong. Apparently, that erroneous conclusion is typically drawn by many conventional treatment practitioners.

Most medical schools do not emphasize diet and nutrition in the treatment of diseases, and there is little emphasis on it within the conventional oncology field.

"The scientific consensus is that cancer cachexia results primarily from an underlying metabolic imbalance induced by the cancer, causing the body's metabolism to speed up," explains Dr. Keith Block, Medical Director of the Block Center for Integrative Cancer Treatment in Evanston, Illinois. "The malignancy generates the production of low-grade inflammatory molecules that break down lean muscle and can disrupt the immune function. The heavy consumption of fats, refined flours, and sugars found in the traditional American diet can increase the inflammation, contributing to a lack of appetite, cause more debilitating weight loss, and actually worsen the very disease the patient is trying to fight." (PR Web 2008)

Dr. Block recently co-authored with Robert Newman, Ph.D., of M.D. Anderson Cancer Center, a study of 1500 chemotherapy patients. The study found that taking antioxidant supplements with chemotherapy had no negative effect on the therapy and might actually increase survival rates, tumor shrinkage, and the patient's ability to tolerate the treatment.

In his popular book, *Beating Cancer with Nutrition*, Patrick Quillin, Ph.D., states that over 40% of cancer patients actually die from malnutrition, not from the cancer. He concluded from his studies that physicians rarely include nutritional counsel in their treatment of cancer patients. The fact is that the cancer itself, as well as the chemotherapy and radiation treatments, suppresses the metabolism process and the appetite resulting in starvation of the whole body including the immune system (Quillin 1998).

According to ABC News medical contributor and nationally renowned authority on nutrition, Dr. David Katz, "Cancer may kill, in part, by causing starvation and conventional therapies may actually exacerbate this aspect of the disease. While these treatments can effectively attack the cancer, they may kill the patient in the process of doing so." Katz, also Associate Professor of Public Health and director of the Prevention Research Center at Yale University further says, "There is thus a need to combine effective assaults on cancer with effective nurturing and nourishing of the body." (PR Web 2008)

In an early 1990's non-randomized clinical trial, Drs. Abram Hoffer and Linus Pauling provided a group of patients with similar cancer a diet of unprocessed food, low in fat, dairy products, and sugar, coupled with therapeutic doses of vitamins and minerals. A control group did not receive the supplemental nutrition support. Of the nutrition program group, 20% lived an average of ten months, 48% lived 72 months, and 32% lived over 10 years with many alive at the end of the study. The entire control group lived an average of only six months.

These references are just a few examples of the great potential of natural dietary and nutritional options for combating cancer. Their potential is made public by medical professionals in the United States only because they can be advocated and prescribed as complements to conventional treatments. I support the advancements in integrating diet and nutrition protocols into conventional treatment. The pursuit by leading integrative oncologists of these advancements has commanded much attention in medical conferences, journals, and organizations. I must ask why the same options shouldn't at least be examined as potentially exclusive treatments that might prove capable against some cancers without being combined with conventional treatments. The answer is obvious and unfortunate. Under our country's current professional and governmental limitations, physicians are not prepared or allowed to initially prescribe any natural dietetic or nutritional treatments as exclusive therapy. So, our research centers and institutions would be wasting valuable time and resources to examine any nutritional treatment as an exclusive option. I believe this position could cause us to overlook something potentially beneficial to the war effort. Nonetheless, I won't die on that hill. Integrating structured nutrition protocols with conventional therapy is a very worthy goal for now.

Food Supplements

Before chemical medications were being developed in laboratories, our ancestors were practicing botanical and mineral medicine for whatever ailed them. Even when they weren't sick, they were eating what we later learned were anti-cancer herbs and spices. No doubt the cancer epidemic we are experiencing today has a lot to do with the toxins our stomach, lungs, and skin ingest. However, the damage the toxins are allowed to do is worsened by the nutritionally impotent and tainted food we eat. The diet of our ancestors included the natural properties that helped keep their incidence of cancer well below what we presently suffer. We can give our bodies the benefit of the natural cancer prevention and healing that previous generations enjoyed. Supplemental nutrients, especially those with anti-cancer properties, are extremely helpful for cancer patients when taken according to the advice and counsel of medical professionals.

Dr. Patrick Quillin refers to the "window of efficacy" for vitamins, herbs, and minerals. Conventional drugs usually have harmful side effects when taken in doses too high and are ineffective when taken in doses too low. The window of efficacy between too high and too low is very narrow. Almost all natural supplements, however, have a very wide window of efficacy. That means relatively high doses can be taken with little risk of harm and some benefit is realized from the smallest doses. Although natural supplements have various levels of side effects, most are unlikely to harm.

Vitamins

This window of efficacy certainly applies to most vitamins not taken in combination with prescription drugs. Research conducted by Dr. Adrienne Bendich and published by the New York Academy of Sciences (Table 5-1) concluded the following (Quillin 2008):

Table 5-1   Window of Efficacy for Vitamins

Supplement	Max Amount	Daily Values	Times Daily Values	Safe Duration
Vitamin A	500,000 iu	5,000 iu	100	Unlimited
Beta-carotene	300,000 iu	None	NA	Extended
Vitamin B-6	500 mg	2 mg	250	6 years
Vitamin C	10,000 mg	60 mg	167	Unlimited
Vitamin E	3,000 mg	30 mg	100	Prolonged
Niacin	6,000 mg	20 mg	300	Unlimited

Let's review some of the more common vitamins purchased over-the-counter (OTC) as they apply to use by cancer patients.

Vitamin A

Vitamin A was the first micronutrient to be acknowledged as having a cancer prevention quality. All known properties of vitamin A directly or indirectly benefit the cancer patient. Vitamin A supplements as the sole therapy in patients with surgery prohibitive lung cancer measurably improved immune functions and tumor responses as reported in a respected German research journal (Micksche 1978). In another study, high doses of vitamin A reduced potentially cancerous mouth cells by 96% (Stich 1991).

Some medical experts warn against the toxicity of high doses of vitamin A that would be required by cancer patients. While vitamin A is probably the most toxic of the most popular supplements, there is plenty of evidence that it is safe, particularly in comparison to its potential benefit. Many European cancer clinics administer up to 2.5 million international units (IU's) per day of emulsified vitamin A for several months with no cause for concern. Of course, dosages at these levels must be under the supervision of medical professionals, but they illustrate the relative safety of the vitamin.

Often, beta-carotene and vitamin A are viewed as being synonymous. Beta-carotene is a form of vitamin A, but has exclusive advantages for cancer prevention and treatment. Beta-carotene in the body takes on a host of responsibilities to ensure that cancer cells are not allowed to develop. It protects the immune cells, inhibits the initial dividing of cancerous cells, and acts as a barrier against carcinogens. Once cancer has initiated, beta-carotene, as a powerful antioxidant, is believed to slow or stop the growth of oxygen-burning cancer cells. Recent research has highlighted the negative side of beta-carotene as a cancer cell catalyst, especially in smokers with lung cancer. The jury is still out on the risk versus benefit of beta-carotene, but cancer cells are certainly sensitive to the nutrient, thereby making it worthy of further study.

Vitamin C

Vitamin C, or ascorbate, has been the focus of numerous cancer prevention and treatment studies. Most medical doctors, naturopaths, and nutritionists agree that vitamin C has strong protective effects against the formation and growth of cancer cells. Balz Frei, Ph.D., Professor of Biochemistry and Biophysics at Oregon State University, explains that vitamin C neutralizes free radicals, harmful molecules in the body that can be produced during chemical reactions that involve oxygen. Free radicals can be the result of exposure to cancer-producing chemicals and other impurities. Vitamin C also helps maintain a healthy immune system for fighting cancer.

Linus Pauling, Ph.D., who won a Nobel Prize for Chemistry and later one for Peace, was probably the world's greatest advocate for vitamin C. One of his several books, *Cancer and Vitamin C*, detailed the multifaceted role of the supplement in combating cancer. Although criticized by physicians and physicians' organizations, he founded the Linus Pauling Institute of Science and Medicine to conduct research in the use of nutrition for preventing and curing degenerative diseases including cancer. Affirmed by his experiments, he maintained that these diseases increased the need for vitamin C considerably above the established required daily amount. Until his death in 1994, Dr. Pauling insisted that vitamin C was a keystone in the war against cancer. Studies at the Mayo Clinic were professed to disprove Pauling's findings on vitamin C. Those studies were controversial and polarized many researches as pro vitamin C or anti vitamin C. Those supporting Pauling's claims dismissed the Mayo studies as scientifically biased.

In 1990, the National Institutes of Health (NIH) hosted a conference on "Vitamin C and Cancer," which confirmed Dr. Pauling's basic findings. However, research of the NIH literature today reveals little support for the vitamin in cancer treatment. The NIH does, however, acknowledge C's benefit in enhancing the immune system and in battling free radicals. It also accepts using vitamin C in large doses, since it is not fat soluble and is non-toxic. Pauling later wrote and spoke profusely on how vitamin C might improve the outcome of cancer patients in treatment. He touted its ability to prevent cancer from breaking down connective tissue for metastasis, its tendency to encapsulate the tumor, its strengthening of the immune system, and its role in hormonal balance.

A most recent Physicians Health Study funded by the NIH concluded that neither vitamin C nor E in pill form help prevent cancer in men. This eight-year study involving over 14,000 male doctors, 50 and over, did not deny the efficacy of these antioxidants obtained through vegetables, fruits, and whole grains. It also did not address the potential benefit of the vitamin administered intravenously. Furthermore, the study did not test the possible benefits of the supplements for warding off other diseases. It simply found that the benefits of these vitamins in preventing cancer may not be realized when the nutrients are received through a supplemental pill. The overwhelming evidence continues to show that antioxidants, including vitamins C, have significant potential to counter the formation and growth of cancer cells. The ACS recommends getting these and other nutrients by eating mostly a variety of plants and grains.

In spite of being somewhat controversial, vitamin C has been shown in numerous studies to be deadly to cancer cells while not harming normal cells. When researchers took leukemia cells from 28 patients and cultured them with vitamin C, 25% of the cultures were inhibited by at least 79% (Park 1980). In animals with implanted tumors, vitamins C and B_{12} together provided for significant tumor regression and 50% survival of the treated group while all of the animals not receiving C and B_{12} died by the 19th day (Poydock 1991). Vitamins

C and B_{12} in combination seemed to selectively shut down tumor growth while helping normal cells flourish.

A recent NCI Cancer Bulletin highlighted new research involving the injection of high doses of vitamin C into mice with aggressive cancers (NCI 2008). The injections slowed the growth of their tumors significantly without affecting normal tissues. The *Proceedings of the National Academy of Sciences* stated that the new findings provide "a firm basis" for advancing vitamin C as a pharmacologic agent for treating human cancer. Study co-author, Dr. Mark Levine, chief of the National Institutes of Health's Molecular and Clinical Nutrition Section, said that Vitamin C was previously thought of as a nutrient, but now it could possibly be used as a drug for treating some cancers. The delivery method seemed to make the difference. Taken orally, ascorbate is limited to a relatively narrow range in the blood. This possibly explains why previous NCI-sponsored clinical trials and the most recent NIH study found no significant benefit from vitamin C given orally. Dr. Len Lichtenfeld, deputy chief medical officer of the ACS, was quick to caution that Vitamin C has a long way to go from theory in the lab to practical application in the clinic. As in most discoveries that excite the integrative oncology enthusiasts, this one will be slow in acceptance by the conventional medicine traditionalists. The Cancer Bulletin notes that scientific interest in vitamin C diminished after the second study in 1985, although many integrative practitioners continued to administer high doses to cancer patients. So, for over two decades, conventional medicine has generally rejected vitamin C while many serious integrative practitioners continue its use. Now the NCI is apparently coming around to acknowledge its value for cancer patients. Wonder what else we are overlooking?

One of the greatest health hazards to ancient sea voyagers was scurvy, an immune system destroyer caused by a long-term deficiency of vitamin C. After centuries of travel on the high seas, the eating of citrus fruits was found to prevent the killer disease. In 1747, the English physician, James Lind, discovered that citrus acid found in limes were a cure for scurvy. Not until over 50 years after the discovery of the citrus fruit remedy did the crews begin carrying citrus fruits on their voyages. The time lags cost thousands of sailors their lives. We have to wonder whether something as simple as vitamin C in certain doses or compounds is lying out there somewhere just waiting to be discovered as a viable cancer treatment.

Vitamin E

Vitamin E is considered by many medical professionals to be the most important of all cancer fighting vitamins. It helps to protect the structure and strength of cells and stimulates the immune function. It also protects healthy cells against toxins and radiation while enhancing the ability of radiation therapy to kill cancer cells. A form of vitamin E selectively attacks cancer cells. One study noted a definite ability of vitamin E to protect laboratory animals from cancer carcinogens (Cook 1980), while another study showed that vitamin E injected into animal tumors significantly reduced or completely eliminated the tumors (Shklar 1987).

As with vitamin C, a recent study concluded that vitamin E seemed to be of little benefit in preventing cancer when taken in pill form. However, the study did not address the benefit of the vitamins from natural diet sources or other forms of intake.

One animal study found that vitamin E increased the effectiveness of a leading chemotherapy drug, 5-FU, against colon cancer in mice (Bruss 2000). Further studies are necessary to determine if the results apply to humans. The statement, "further studies are necessary," is a recurring disclaimer in the debate over natural nutritional supplements. Something shows promise in animal or laboratory studies, but "further studies are necessary." Who's going to do these studies when medical professionals are not interested, medical schools can't afford them, pharmaceutical companies get little return on investment from them, and the government is obligated to the pharmaceutical companies? Animal experiments are cheap; human studies are extremely expensive. The answer is that there will be no such studies unless there are organized, grass roots efforts to fund them and demand them.

Laboratory tests have revealed that, when vitamin E is combined with succinic acid, it becomes a powerful agent for interrupting the growth of cancer cells without disturbing healthy cells. Various kinds of laboratory cultured cancerous cell and tumors have been destroyed or their growth inhibited by this vitamin E succinate compound.

In addition to its potential for arresting cancer growth directly, indications are that vitamin E can be a remedy to hair loss associated with conventional cancer treatment. According to a study highlighted in the *New England Journal of Medicine*, 69% of patients on Adriamicin, a common chemotherapy prescription that is usually accompanied by hair loss, did not experience the hair loss while taking structured levels of vitamin E. Those who did lose some of their hair were believed to have received the vitamin E too late in the study process (Wood 1985). Hair loss during cancer treatment is one of the worst side effects that patients have to tolerate. If vitamin E has been shown to be a potential means of avoiding this psychologically debilitating aspect of treatment, and if the nutrient is assuredly safe, why has more research not been done to verify its utility? Here is a natural, low-cost supplement that preliminary studies have shown to have significant cancer fighting properties and one that has the possibly of reducing an agonizing side effect of cancer treatment. Yet, serious studies of its potential by recognized research institutions are not even being considered.

One of the frustrations of integrative therapy advocates is that many studies to determine whether certain dietary supplements are effective against cancer result in positive findings, but the studies don't continue into observable clinical trials. Further testing is awaiting someone who is interested and has the resources.

Herbals

Over 20,000 different chemical compounds assist plants in their growth and protect them from harm. These compounds, called "bioflavonoids" or sometimes just "flavonoids," support the photosynthesis process and guard the plants from the sun's radiation and other dangers. Bioflavonoids are widely distributed in all plant life producing bright color pigmentation while protecting the plant cells from everything from microbes to insects. They are not technically vitamins, but are sometimes referred to as vitamin P. They are scavengers of free radical cells that are precursors to cancer cells. Because the body does not produce bioflavonoids, they must be supplied through the diet or supplementation.

The greatest concentrations of bioflavonoids are found in deep, dark colored vegetables and fruits. One type of bioflavonoid is prevalent in black grapes, beets, red onions, and most berries. Another type is in cranberries and raspberries. Several types are present in kale, spinach, apples, green tea, black tea, green beans, and citrus fruits. The life-supporting and protective qualities of bioflavonoids in plants have been found, through the ages, to produce the same qualities in animals.

In laboratory experiments, animals with implanted tumors lived longer when given bioflavonoids from grape rinds (Kolde 1996). Bioflavonoids administered in the diet of rats helped to reduce DNA damage from certain carcinogens (LeBon 1992). In other studies, various bioflavonoids have produced striking reductions in animal cancers, often up to almost complete cessation of tumor growth (Wattenberg 1970).

It is a very small step in deductive reasoning to conclude that the bioflavonoids created to energize and protect plants are also created to benefit animals, particularly humans, through nutritional intake of those plants. From ancient civilizations up to recent generations, people have relied on selected plants with healing properties to cure all kinds of ailments and diseases. The typical diets of previous generations included much more bioflavonoid-rich plant content than today's diets. The sharp reduction of these plants in our modern diet may contribute to cancer's free reign in our bodies. Once cancer attacks, the lack of sufficient bioflavonoids in our system may be frustrating our body's ability to fight it. What if the principal reason that there is so much more cancer today than in previous centuries has to do with our avoidance of bioflavonoids? What if the cancers that attacked previous generations were in large measure contained by diets rich in bioflavonoids? How much decisive research is being done to determine how cancer patients could benefit from bioflavonoids? The answer to the last question is obviously almost none.

Several herbal foods with high concentrations of bioflavonoids are recommended by nutritionists and naturopathic doctors for cancer prevention and as supplements during cancer treatment. Of course, any supplement or supplemental food should only be used in coordination with the cancer treatment physician.

Curcumin

Curcumin produces the bright yellow pigment in turmeric, a flavoring agent in curry spice. It is found in most mustards. It helps the immune system by protecting immune cells from their own poisons (pro-oxidants). In animal experiments, curcumin has been shown to be directly toxic to tumor cells (Kuttan 1985). Turmeric with curcumin has provided significant reduction in skin cancer lesions for patients who have failed therapy with chemo, radiation, and surgery (Kuttan 1987).

Frankincense

Frankincense is a familiar term to most of us as one of the three gifts brought by the Wise Men to baby Jesus. It is now being evaluated for its possible benefit to cancer patients. The compound (resin from the Boswellia tree) causes no major adverse effects and is safe for human consumption and long-term use (Washington Post 2008). The NCI Cancer Bulletin recently highlighted a clinical trial being conducted by the Cleveland Clinic Taussig Cancer Center which is testing dietary and herbal therapy for brain cancer. The Phase II study is testing frankincense as part of a vegan diet for patients with high-grade Gliomas, a type of aggressive brain tumor. Frankincense has been touted for centuries in some cultures as a healing agent for various diseases. It has been shown in animal and human studies to reduce inflammation, particularly in osteoarthritis patients. Laboratory studies have suggested that it may also cause human brain cancer cells to undergo programmed cell death (apoptosis). Dr. Glen Stevens, Principal Investigator for this clinical trial said, "Some small studies have suggested that frankincense extract may help limit brain edema and even have an anti-tumor effect. Let's hope that dietary changes in conjunction with use of this herbal preparation will help improve patient outcomes and act in a complementary fashion with standard treatments for high-grade Gliomas."

Garlic

Garlic, written about as a medicine over 6000 years ago, was one of the contents of Egyptian King Tutankhamen's tomb. Records show that slaves who built the Great Pyramids relied on garlic for increased energy. Hippocrates, the father of modern medicine, used garlic to heal infections and reduce pain. In just the last few decades, over 2000 scientific studies have proven what our ancient ancestors knew—the healing value of garlic. Research is now showing that garlic may impact cancer by inhibiting carcinogen formation in the body. It appears to interfere with the transformation of normal cells to pre-cancerous cells (Wargovich 1992). It also seems to prevent the formation of blood vessels in tumor masses (anti-angiogenesis). In one animal study, garlic was more effective than the main drug used in human bladder cancer (Marsh 1987). Extensive review of the literature shows impressive and multiple ways that garlic can help the cancer patient. It deserves further study. The ACS's Guide to Complementary and Alternative Methods states that laboratory studies suggest garlic may be of benefit in reducing tumor growth. It has been shown to kill human colon cancer cells in mice. Again, the disclaimer is that human testing is needed (Bruss 2000).

Ginseng

Ginseng was used by Chinese physicians several thousand years ago to treat almost every illness imaginable. Today, we are learning that the confidence these ancient physicians had in this herb may have been well placed. Initial clinical studies of Ginseng's potential anticancer characteristics have been inconclusive perhaps because differences in the herb are so wide-ranging. Concentrations of cancer fighting properties vary depending on the type, place of origin, processing procedures, and distribution techniques. All ginseng products need to be studied. Tests have shown that ginseng stimulates the immune system to produce more macrophages (cells that literally eat cancer cells and harmful cellular debris) (Jie 1984). One study showed a 75% reduction in average tumor size in mice after just eight days of ginseng intake (Hau 1990). Ginseng also slowed tumor growth and lengthened survival in rats with chemically-induced liver cancer (Li 1991). Obviously, much more clinical study needs to be dedicated to this very promising anticancer herb.

Green Tea

Green Tea is processed from the Camellia sinensis plant. The antioxidants found in tea (catechins) appear to selectively inhibit the growth of cancer. The catechins are released abundantly in green tea, whereas they are almost negligible in black tea. Steaming the leaves produces green tea, while drying the leaves produces black tea. Apparently, the drying process reduced the catechins. Although, the most potent anticancer properties come from green tea, it only accounts for 20% of tea consumed worldwide. The National Cancer Institutes of China and Japan have been researching green tea with the same fervor that the American NCI has been researching chemotherapy drugs (Quillin 1998). However, in recent years, green tea has been getting the attention of our own NCI. Its research is showing that tea catechins scavenge oxidants before cell injuries occur, reduce the incidence and size of chemically induced tumors, and inhibit the growth of tumor cells (Dufresne 2008). Ongoing NCI studies are testing green tea's effect against skin cancer. The prospective use of green tea to help prevent and treat cancer tumors certainly deserves the increased priorities of the NCI and other research-supporting institutions in America.

Silymarin

Silymarin, or milk thistle, is a liver detoxifier, a tissue regenerator, and an augmenter of the immune system. It is widely prescribed in Europe for liver diseases. Since the liver is the main organ involved in removing toxins from the body, its health is essential to the body's cancer battle. The liver also stores most vitamins and minerals as well as produces bile for digestion. It is one of the fronts in the complementary therapy fight against cancer. Silymarin has also been shown in tests to heal damaged liver tissue and to protect liver cells (Werbach 1994).

Minerals

There are 22 minerals that are considered essential to bodily functions. They are particularly critical to cancer patients for two reasons. First, some of the minerals have qualities that help in the body's fight against the disease. Second, the effects of cancer often cause shortages of vital minerals. When the cancer patient needs them most, minerals are often reduced by the cancer.

Cancer usually causes the following conditions which lead to mineral deficiency:

- Loss of appetite and a poor selection of foods
- Decreased mineral absorption due to conventional treatment
- Decreased potency of minerals due to drug interactions
- Loss of minerals due to diarrhea and vomiting
- More minerals required due to tumor growth

Seven minerals are needed by the body in relatively large amounts: calcium, phosphorus, magnesium, sulfur, sodium, potassium, and chloride. Although these minerals are important to balancing the body's nutrition, they don't appear at present to contribute directly to fighting cancer. Trace minerals, on the other hand are needed by the body in relatively small amounts, but have a more direct impact on cancer.

Zinc and Copper

Zinc and copper, both trace minerals, play a similar, but important, role in the immune system. Cancer patients may need to supplement zinc and copper levels that have been depleted in their systems. Zinc and copper enhance T cell and Natural Killer (NK) cell activity necessary for optimum operation of the immune system. Low zinc levels have been linked to increased size of head or neck tumors, more advanced stages of disease, and a greater number of unplanned hospitalizations. Copper complexes have shown to have anti-cancer properties in laboratory studies (Bruss 2000). If zinc and copper are so essential to keeping immune cells healthy and keeping tumor size small, more study is needed regarding these minerals as major cancer fighting agents.

Selenium

Selenium, according to researchers Maureen Keane and Daniella Chace in their book, *What to Eat if You Have Cancer*, has been shown in animal studies to inhibit the formation of tumors and may slow their growth. It helps the body defend against free radicals. There is also evidence that it may be directly toxic to tumors. As with most trace minerals, selenium is found naturally in foods such as certain fish, barley, brown rice, and sunflower seeds. The *ACS's Guide to Complementary and Alternative Cancer Methods* affirms selenium as a nutrient that may prevent the development and progression of cancer. Both animal and human studies suggest that selenium may play a role in lowering a person's risk of developing cancer, and reducing death rates from cancer in those who already have the disease (Bruss 2000). Since selenium appears to be directly toxic to tumors, maybe researchers should be subjecting it to more laboratory scrutiny. Imagine something as natural and harmless as a trace mineral being discovered by medical science as a significant breakthrough in cancer treatment.

Bovine Cartilage

Approximately 50 nutrients are considered essentials for our diet. However, there are thousands more that have been discovered to be necessary for optimal health. These "accessory" nutrients found in a variety of common and not-so-common foods are gaining increased interest, especially for use with cancer patients. One such accessory is animal cartilage. Bovine, or cow, cartilage got the attention of some researchers about a half-century ago. Dr. John Prudden, a Harvard degreed MD, was professor of surgery at Columbia-Presbyterian Medical Center in New York in the 1950's. Dr. Prudden treated a 70 year old, hopeless stage IV breast cancer patient with the bovine cartilage. Bovine tracheal cartilage, or BTC, was administrated topically and through injection. The cancer was healed completely. Prudden conducted $7 million in research in BTC and was awarded a patent for it in 1962.

In the 1980's, William Lane, PhD, experimented with shark cartilage in anti-angiogenesis therapy. Recall from the discussion of garlic that anti-angiogenesis is the prevention of blood vessels from forming around a tumor, thus shutting down the tumor's lifeline of blood. Dr. Lane's book, *Sharks Don't Get Cancer*, started the use of shark cartilage as a major nutrition option among complementary cancer therapies. The belief was that cartilage, especially from sharks, starved tumor cells to death by taking away the vessels that sustained them. The cartilage theories were simultaneously being affirmed by the works of Dr. Robert Langer of MIT and Dr. Judah Folkman of Harvard who published a work indicating that cartilage can, in fact, stop angiogenesis in cultured tumors. Langer's subsequent research found that tumors were limited in growth to 1 to 2 centimeters without growing blood vessels (angiogenesis) to support their expansion. Further study by Folkman demonstrated that, when normal cell growth turned to rapid and uncontrolled tumor growth, the angiogenesis process sped up tremendously. Later Harvard research reported a pronounced link between angiogenesis and tumor growth.

Dr. Folkman's landmark work in anti-angiogenesis began when he was chief of surgery at Boston's Children's Hospital. Many scientists predict that, when a successful treatment for cancer is finally found, it will be built on the work of Dr. Folkman. A peer-reviewed article by Dr. Prudden analyzed 31 human terminal cancer patients followed for 15 years. Eleven, or 35% of the patients, were cured using 9 grams daily of oral bovine tracheal cartilage as the sole therapy. Seventeen, or 55%, showed some benefit then relapsed, and three, or 10% showed no improvement (Quillin 1998).

So, the cumulative studies of Dr. Prudden, Dr. Lane, Dr. Langer, and Dr. Folkman, as well as many of their colleagues strongly support the case that bovine (BTC) and shark cartilage have been found to slow or kill cancer tumors by anti-angiogenesis. To quote Dr. Patrick Quillen, "Of all the impressive healing agents in nature's "pharmacy," none is more safe, cost-effective, versatile, and promising than BTC." The NCI has shown some interest in further cartilage research in their labs. Preclinical trials have shown promise, especially in the anti-angiogenesis factor. Few actual clinical trials have been conducted, and those that have appear to be inconclusive. It remains high on the list of integrative medicine experts as worthy of further study.

The Debate

Only a few representative samples of nutritional augmenters for cancer treatment have been showcased here. This field of research is almost unlimited in potential findings. The debate is unending as to the type, amount, and balance of nutrition and supplements that are necessary to fight the cancer battle. The philosophies range from not getting all worked up over food to total vegetarian diets to mega doses of supplements. Some believe what cancer patients eat doesn't matter, while others are convinced that what they eat will cure their cancer. Most scientific evidence falls on the side of nutrition having a substantial role in preventing cancer and a potential role in treating it. Minor studies, trials, and anecdotal evidence show that there is significant potential for nutritional components to slow or reverse cancer's attack. What is missing is aggressive effort by large, respected medical science institutions to conduct controlled clinical trials for nutrition-based theories. Only recently have health professionals paid serious attention to nutrition in the <u>prevention</u> of cancer. That attention, along with the socio-economic movement it has produced, has benefited each of us. The same level of attention to nutrition for the <u>treatment</u> of cancer is well overdue. I sincerely believe that nutrition as an integral part of cancer treatment, and in rare cases perhaps as the exclusive treatment, can revolutionize our whole approach to the war on cancer.

The present Catch 22 is that only a meager number of oncologists have the education, training, and experience to administer or even recommend nutritional complements to conventional therapy. Complementary nutritional therapy will not be widely used until it is available and acceptable on a broad scale. The few integrative oncologists that practice nutritional therapy must be sought out by more patients, thus creating a demand for it that exceeds supply. Doctors are business people, too, and many will rise to the need by becoming qualified in integrative oncology. The new strategy for the war on cancer requires such a tremendous expansion in this specialty field.

CHAPTER 6

THE PROMISE OF NEW METHODS

In addition to the proven and potential benefits from diet and nutrition, new and exciting natural methodologies abound for cancer treatment application. Many of these methodologies are being approved and used in whole or in part with success, but need more refined testing in order to play an expanded role in the treatment process.

High Potential Procedural Complementary Therapies

Several procedures, some old and some new, are drawing the attention of cancer researchers and treatment practitioners. These have received a significant amount of testing and are being practiced in some venues.

Anti-angiogenesis

I have referenced anti-angiogenesis previously as having great potential for cancer treatment. So, let's look at it a little more closely. Since 85 percent of all cancer deaths are from tumors, new therapies that target tumors get the majority of research attention. Anti-angiogenesis therapy has not yet proven itself to be effective in all types and levels of cancer tumors. But, it is becoming generally accepted as an advantageous complement to conventional treatment.

In 1971, Dr. Judah Folkman's research hypothesized that tumor growth is angiogenesis dependent, meaning the errant cells have to generate their own blood supply system in order to stay alive and grow. As is typical for new tactics in the cancer war, the gears turned very slowly in testing and acceptance of the idea. It was not until some 20 years later that angiogenesis inhibitors were used successfully against a human tumor. In 1999, anti-angiogenesis theories became a top priority for the NCI. Clinical trials combining angiogenesis inhibitors with toxic treatment have led to documented increases in survival rates. However, use of angiogenesis as the sole treatment (monotherapy) has not been sufficiently tested (Davis, Herbst, and Abbruzzese 2008).

Anti-angiogenesis can target the cancer cells both directly and indirectly. Direct angiogenesis inhibitors block vascular cell production, thus disallowing the tumors to generate a viable blood system. Indirect angiogenesis inhibitors target and block tumor cell proteins that control the tumor's ability to generate its own vascular system. The methodology depends on the type of cancer, and both tactics can severely restrict the cancer cells' ability to grow.

Presently, anti-angiogenesis studies and clinical trials are pursuing the weakening of tumor cells which allows conventional treatment to be more effective with less potency and toxicity. We may be witnessing the development of one of the most beneficial combinations of complementary and conventional treatments ever. We would hope that, as these trials progress, we would see more anti-angiogenesis and less toxicity in the mix. This is another case where virtually harmless complementary therapy could reduce the level and duration of chemotherapy needed. Utopia would be the inhibitors blocking tumor growth completely when applied as a monotherapy. Logic and experience would convince us that it will never happen. We must remember, though, that established medicine said initially that Dr. Folkman's basic anti-angiogenesis hypothesis was flawed. A lesson we seem to consistently find difficult to learn is to not reject any potential cancer option outright until it has run its course in the scientific research system. Even having proven itself in the system, anti-angiogenesis, like many of its unconventional predecessors, is still having some difficulty getting traction in mainstream cancer treatment.

Gene Testing and Therapy

When we think of genetics in connection with cancer, we usually think of individual genetic proclivity to develop the disease. Genetic testing to assess the risk of cancer is a relative new concept, but one that is getting a lot of attention and needs much more study. Less news making, but equally important is gene therapy to reduce or eliminate the cancer once it is established. This also has immeasurable possibilities for advancing the war on cancer.

DNA is a vast chemical information database in the nucleus of every cell. Each nucleus contains chromosomes, or DNA molecules. Each DNA molecule contains genes within a structure of two long, spiraled strands made of millions of chemical building blocks called bases. There are only four chemical bases, but they are arranged in almost unlimited combinations. The order of these arrangements conveys messages much like the alphabet forms words, sentences, and entire books. Every cell in a particular body contains the same DNA. Thus, from conception until death, our DNA commands each of our cells, and therefore our bodies, to form our appearance, personality, basic health, intelligence, psychological make-up, and even our actions to a degree. However, chromosome genes in DNA molecules give cells different roles. A brain cell is directed to be different from a bone cell, for instance.

A healthy body depends on the interactions of thousands of gene proteins in perfect harmony. More than 4000 diseases stem from less than harmonious altered genes inherited from one's mother or father and ultimately from one's ancestors (NCI 2008). A propensity for certain types of cancers can often be determined by an individual's genes. This is currently a rapidly developing science.

Mistakes constantly occur in everyone's DNA, but healthy cells can almost always repair the damage. Unfortunately, if repair mechanisms fail, mutations can be passed on to future cells. Although all cancer is technically genetic, less than 10% is actually directly inherited. Most cancers start with random cell mutations from uncorrected mistakes or environmental agents such as radiation or chemicals (NCI 2008). Yet, wayward DNA, inherited or acquired, can be occasionally passed on to offspring. Therefore, genetic testing of an individual relative to family history of cancer can sometimes help assess the risk of developing the disease and provide prevention opportunities. Somewhat more challenging, but presently showing progress is the study of managing genetic processes in the treatment of cancer.

Identifying genes associated with disease involves tracking every chemical base in each of the 25,000 genes as well as the spaces between them. This identification process is called "mapping the human genome." This colossal task was only recently accomplished by an international collaboration known as the Human Genome Project. This project has opened up a whole new realm of possibilities in both the prevention and treatment of cancer.

Researchers are presently experimenting with the introduction of tumor suppressor genes, or antioncogenes, into rapidly dividing cells to slow down or arrest tumor growth. Viruses which cannot reproduce are the transport of choice to the tumor location, thereby reducing the risk of normal cells being damaged by another type of virus that reproduces itself. The virus is genetically engineered by infusing it with the suppression gene. The virus infects the tumor and deposits the suppression gene which goes to work dismantling the genetic structure of the tumor cells. This invading gene causes damage to tumor cell genes essential for cell growth and division. If successful, this would leave the tumor cells dormant or dead.

A subset of gene therapy for cancer is anti-telomerase therapy. Telomerase is an enzyme that adds specific DNA functions to chromosomes, extending their telomeres (life cycle regulators). The enzyme can promote cancer cells by allowing them to bypass the normal cell life cycle and become "immortal." They divide virtually forever in the form of growing tumors. Healthy tissues contain little if any telomerase. It seems to be mostly present in genetically damaged tissues. Telomerase activity has been observed in 90% of all human tumors, suggesting that the immortality made possible by the enzyme is key to cancer development. A number of research groups have experimented with the use of telomerase inhibitors in animals. Phase I and II human clinical trials began in 2006. Expediting these trials would likely be of tremendous value to integrative practitioners, since it could reduce some necessity for conventional therapies.

Monoclonal Antibody Therapy

Monoclonal antibody therapy is a type of passive immunotherapy and most often used without chemotherapy or radiation. After a decade of use, it has proven to have few side effects. Any side effects during the initial adjustment period are relatively mild. Large amounts of antibodies made in the lab are injected into the cancer patient. The antibodies create a powerful immunity force with a two-fold objective: to attack the malignant cells and to block specific tumor cell receptors.

Frequently, tumor cells are not recognized by the patient's immune natural system because they are not differentiated enough from his or her normal cells. An immune system super-activated by monoclonal antibodies tends to be more successful at finding the unusual antigens that are recognized as inappropriate for the cell type and fight them aggressively.

Some tumor cells display cell surface receptors that are rare or absent on the surfaces of healthy cells. These receptors activate pathways for unregulated growth and cell division. Monoclonal antibodies are designed to destroy the specific antigens on the surfaces of tumors that support the tumor receptors.

Monoclonal antibody therapy has proven itself worthy of broader-scale use and more serious application to cancers. A small number of non-substantial inadequacies still need to be resolved. The more it can be perfected, the less burden patients will have to bear with chemotherapy and radiation.

Vaccine Therapy

The campaign in recent years to encourage young women to be vaccinated with human papillomavirus (HPV) to help prevent cervical cancer has raised awareness to vaccines as a hope for the future of cancer prevention. Numerous types of cancer, including cervical cancer, have a virus as their source. In 2006, HPV vaccine was approved as the first vaccine in the United States to be developed for a known risk factor for cancer. We certainly need to continue a full-scale effort toward prevention options in the exploration of vaccines.

However, vaccine solutions should also be persistently sought in the treatment of existing cancers.

The Vaccine Branch of the NCI's Center for Cancer Research has engineered a vaccine that shows great promise in eradicating some advanced breast cancer tumors in mice. The results of the study were released in March, 2008. This new therapeutic vaccine is designed to stimulate the body's immune system so that it recognizes cancer as an invader in specific tissues. It uses a modified virus to seek out a surface receptor prevalent in one out of four women who have breast cancer. When mice were injected with breast cancer cells and the vaccine simultaneously, no tumors formed. When the vaccine was given after the cancer cells injection, small tumors formed and disappeared in 45 days and did not reappear. Even tumors that were allowed to metastasize to other organs before the vaccine was administered were ultimately completely cleared.

"A vaccine offers several advantages over a monoclonal antibody treatment which targets a single region on a receptor," said Dr. Jay Berzofsky, research team leader, "A vaccine may induce the production of several different antibodies and target multiple regions on a receptor, making it harder for the tumor to mutate and escape the effects of therapy." (NCI 2008)

At the time of this writing, the University of Arkansas for Medical Sciences (UAMS) was initiating clinical trials on a new immunotherapy vaccine for breast cancer. This vaccine mimics antigens that cause the body to produce extra antibodies that target both the vaccine and the cancer cells. The first phase of the trial will involve women with metastatic cancer and those who have relapsed after going into remission.

The Provenge cancer vaccine test results were recently presented to the American Urological Association. Unlike traditional vaccines that prevent disease, Provenge treats cancer by training the immune system to fight tumors. Earlier tests on 127 men with prostate cancer showed an average of 4.5 months longer life for those who were given the vaccine as compared to those who were given a placebo. The latest testing involving 512 men with advanced prostate cancer resulted in even greater survivability. Several scientists have expressed hope that this new approach to fighting cancer will take cancer treatment beyond the surgery, radiation, and chemotherapy almost exclusively used now.

Hyperthermia

Dr. Josef Issels was a 20th century German physician who pioneered a whole-body approach to cancer therapy with emphasis on the body's natural immune system. Although, he didn't dispute conventional practices of surgery and chemotherapy, he believed that the key to curing cancer was to strengthen the weakened immune system that allowed it to happen. He might be considered the father of integrative oncology. His combination of therapies relied heavily on what he called "sweat therapy" or induced hyperthermia. Used for centuries in Europe to treat chronic diseases, it causes a pronounced increase in white blood cell count. The white blood cells are the core of the disease fighting antibodies of the body. Dr. Issels administered monthly "fever shots" to patients which induced a high fever for up to five hours. In 1984, the FDA approved this practice as a valid cancer treatment. Five years later, the NCI stated that heat therapy increases the effectiveness of other treatments by 25 to 35 percent.

BSD Medical, a manufacturer of state-of-the art hyperthermia therapy equipment, sees their mission as overcoming important clinical impediments that handicap the traditional tools for treating cancer. A BSD Medical press release announced that, in phase III clinical trials, when hyperthermia therapy was added to radiation therapy, significant improvements were reported for certain tumors, approximately doubling the rate of tumor response for some cancers. Heat stimulates blood circulation in tumors making radiation treatments more effective while directly killing certain cancer cells. Researchers are currently evaluating the effectiveness of hyperthermia in supporting drug delivery by enlarging tumor pores (BSD Medical 2008).

A recent *Boston Globe* article observed that traditional therapies offer little to help shrink cancerous tumors. The article went on to say that, according to clinical studies, when tumors are treated with radiation therapy and hyperthermia in combination, they tend to shrink, sometimes dramatically (Boston Globe 2008).

Another hyperthermia victory occurred in a recent study published in *Radiotherapy and Oncology*, an official publication of the *European Society for Therapeutic Radiology and Oncology*. Heat treatment by the BSD 2000 machine improved bladder cancer's five-year survival rate by 13 percent. A multi-center trial in Italy reported that bladder surgery patients had a recurrence rate of 57 percent with the Mitomycin-C drug alone, but that rate fell to 17 percent with the addition of hyperthermia therapy. That same trial included patients with cervical or rectal cancer. The treatment resulted in similar successes for all types of cancers. For instance, hyperthermia increased the three-year survival rate for cervical cancer by 26 percent.

Hyperthermia is now common treatment in most European countries and is officially recommended by the German Cancer Society. It has yet to be generally accepted by oncologists in the United States. The BSD 2000 machine is made in the United States but is limited to investigational use by the Food and Drug Administration (Moss 2009).

Just before this book was submitted to the publisher, a breaking news article in the *Journal of the National Cancer Institute* again drew attention to hyperthermia. The article reported that a randomized trial in Europe showed that patients given chemotherapy plus hyperthermia had a median disease-free survival period of almost twice that of those who got chemotherapy alone. Elizabeth Repasky, Ph.D., of Roswell Park Cancer Institute, Buffalo, N.Y., commented on the trial results, "We are on a verge, I think, of a major new adjuvant cancer therapy that will not replace chemotherapy or radiation, but will make them work a lot better." Zeljko Vujaskovic, M.D., Ph.D., a radiation oncologist at Duke University Medical Center, although encouraged by the finding, was skeptical about its impact. He said, "I have been in the field 20 years, and I see how much benefit patients have, but institutions are not willing to use it."

At the very least, intense research needs to continue into hyperthermia as a complement to conventional cancer therapy. In the best scenario, research would test the use of hyperthermia as a stand-alone therapy. Since it has been proven to make tumors more vulnerable to radiation and chemotherapy, would it possibly make the same tumors more vulnerable to the body's natural immune system?

Imagine a detoxified immune system significantly boosted by special diet and nutritional supplements working against tumors weakened by hyperthermia. That combination might be a formidable cancer fighting force.

Although these late-breaking research projects will take some time to move through the pains-taking clinical trial phases, it is exciting news for those of us who are in the race for more palatable and successful tactics for the war strategy. The vaccines should have very little side effects and could be a viable integrative therapy if not someday a replacement for conventional therapy.

Other Complementary Therapies on the Periphery of Science

There is another category of promising weapons for the cancer war arsenal which should receive attention. This category of practices has earned consideration for a place at the integrative oncology table, but has yet to gain a consensus among medical scientists. Some have been researched and officially rejected. Proponents of those question the validity of the research. Others have not had the support for bona fide testing, but claim testimonial proof of authenticity. Some components of some of them are practiced in leading medical institutions throughout America. Therefore, I believe they deserve their day in the court of certified scientific testing as potential cancer therapy. Some of those that have been tested and rejected may deserve an unbiased review by different researchers.

Chelation Therapy

The word *chelation* comes from the Greek root word *chele* which means "to bind." The concept of chelation is to introduce a substance into the body that will bind harmful impurities to itself and remove them through bodily functions. Supporters understand chelation to be a safe and effective way to detoxify the body and free up its immune system to fight cancer. Our typical lifestyle and the environment in which we live cause us to take in harmful substances constantly. Although our immune system normally works very hard to breakdown and remove these impurities, it is a losing battle over time. Our bodies store chemical components within tissues, gases, and blood that harm our cells and pollute our body fluids. Some of these unwelcome guests can cause dysfunctions that lead to illnesses and diseases including cancer. The more we can do to help the immune system, the more it will be relieved to concentrate on disease-causing carcinogens and uncontrolled cells. Chelation therapy usually involves a combination of an amino acid, herbals, and vitamins taken intravenously or orally.

Chelation therapy was first used in 1950 to treat lead poisoning in factory workers. It was highly successful in removing the lead and certain other metals that produced free radicals in the body. Since then, the therapy has been used extensively in alternative and integrative cancer treatment and by naturopaths in cancer prevention protocols. It has yet to find its place in the practices of conventional oncologists. Although chelation is legal in the United States and is a part of many integrative therapy practices, it is still considered outside the mainstream of conventional medicine. Some doctors argue that chelation rids the body of essential bacteria and, therefore, does more harm than good. It seems perfectly logical that any patient being treated for cancer should have his or her body operating at its highest capacity. This would include having the body detoxified as much as possible. Hopefully, chelation will soon be at least an optional study in our medical schools and considered by more physicians.

Laetrile Therapy

Laetrile is the common name of a compound also known as amygdalin. Its nutrition designation is vitamin B_{17}. Bitter almonds, one source of amygdalin, was first used by a Chinese herbalist, Pen T'Sao, in 2800 B.C. Amygdalin is also found in kernels of certain fruit pits including those of apricots, peaches, plums, and cherries. Apricot pits are presently the principal source. Amygdalin was first isolated as a medical compound in 1830 by two French chemists. As researchers began serious pursuit of a cure for cancer in the early 1950's, Ernst Krebs, Jr., an American biochemist synthesized a compound from the apricot kernel. This new compound, evolved from amygdalin, was patented as Laetrile[R]. Later, the capital L was dropped as laetrile became the common name for other similar compounds. Laetrile contains natural cyanide. The anti-cancer concept of laetrile involves the characteristic of malignant cells to produce a particular enzyme not present in normal cells. Laetrile advocates say this cancer cell enzyme releases the cyanide from the laetrile molecule upon contact allowing the cyanide to poison the cancer cell. Conversely, they believe a different enzyme in a normal cell binds the cyanide upon contact with laetrile, neutralizing it, and passing it out of the body through the urine.

Laetrile has had a colorful history to say the least. The conventional medical establishment adamantly opposed it from the beginning. They took immediate issue with cyanide toxicity which laetrile proponents claim is non-existent when it is injected into the body. Several years ago, the FDA conducted a Phase I test that pronounced laetrile nontoxic. Subsequently, over 20 states gave cancer patients the right to choose laetrile for their therapy. Opponents, however, continued to charge that laetrile has been proven ineffective in repeated studies and clinical trials. The NCI subjected laetrile to their clinical trial process, and, in 1981, declared it non effective. Advocates counter that researchers have yet to give it a clinical trial under the same standards and protocols that are used for other drugs. It has been vilified in political proceedings and banned by the courts. Presently, it is illegal to prescribe or sell laetrile in the United States. It continues to be used in many countries and is accepted in various medical cultures around the world as a successful cancer treatment.

The development and use of laetrile has been within a seemingly dark and almost conspiracy-like environment. Initial researchers and practitioners of the product claim to have undeniable proof that it works, but most feel they have been harassed and stifled in their efforts by the medical and pharmaceutical establishment. The American Cancer Society, the American Medical Association, the National Cancer Institute, and other agencies and institutions have been accused of biased studies, legal maneuvering, and slander in organized efforts to refute the legitimacy of laetrile. In Chapter Seven, you will read Dr. Contreras' opinion of the NCI sponsored study which he characterizes as not in keeping with the institute's own standards and procedures. In turn, these respected institutions label laetrile researchers and practitioners as illegitimate if not "quacks." Pharmaceutical giants and defenders of laetrile have been exchanging accusations of conspiracy and protectionism for years. If you ever want to read some drama-in-real-life, just Google "laetrile" and begin an endless review of entertaining, but sad stories.

I don't consider myself a conspiracy theorist. And, I am not convinced enough to resurrect the laetrile controversy as its newest advocate. However, it is interesting that its supporters have taken so much heat. High level effort has gone into ensuring that it is banned from American medical and pharmacy practices. It is still used widely in other parts of the world. What if something natural and cheap from an apricot pit could be proven as effective against some cancers as any chemotherapy drug? Perhaps laetrile deserves more human clinical trials under the utmost standards and procedures of America's most reputable laboratories.

Radio Waves and Nanoparticles

A most recent discovery has developed from a seemingly coincidental merging of particular people and situations. I should add here that I do not believe much of anything in life is coincidental. I am convinced that God ultimately orchestrates all activity in His own strategic timing and method. The account I am about to present is, in my opinion, a miraculous coming together of people and situations that brings yet another bright ray of hope for future cancer victims. It is about a radio wave generator that heats nanoparticles, or nanotubes, injected into cells of cancer tumors.

John Kanzius is not a doctor or scientist. He is a retired radio station owner who knows something about radio technology. After being diagnosed with terminal leukemia, he underwent 36 rounds of chemotherapy. Although very sick throughout his therapy, he stated on the CBS television program *60 Minutes* that it was looking into the hollow eyes of sick children on the cancer ward that really motivated him to try something—anything—that might have a shot at curing cancer. He told *60 Minutes* correspondent Lesley Stahl that, during one of his many sleepless nights, he was overwhelmed with the nagging thought "There's gotta be a better way to treat cancer." So, he went to the kitchen and started what was to become a life-changing project of building a radio wave machine. The machine would target cancer cells and destroy them with microscopic precision. A garage-based laboratory and a $200,000 investment began a quest for cancer cell destruction through extreme heat from radio waves. His early experiments involved injecting hot dogs with copper sulfate as the catalyst to super-heat a cell-defined area. Temperature would rise sharply in the area where the metal solution was without affecting the surrounding area.

Now, the first "coincidence." While being treated at M. D. Anderson Cancer Center in Houston, Kanzius shared his experiment results with Steven Curley, M.D., professor in the Center's Department of Surgical Oncology. Dr. Curley was very impressed with the concept. Both he and Kanzius researched the concept with various materials and techniques of heating cells laden with metals by radio waves.

"This technology may allow us to treat just about any kind of cancer you can imagine," Dr. Curley told Stahl on *60 Minutes*. "I've gotta tell you, in 20 years of research, this is the most exciting thing that I've encountered." (CBS News 2008)

Keep in mind, this is a renowned cancer researcher who has been looking for conventional medicine answers to cancer treatment for 20 years. He said that this relatively simple alternative treatment discovery is "the most exciting thing he has ever seen."

As the research progressed, it became apparent that space-age nanoparticles would have to be used in the cells that received the heat, and they would have to discriminate between tumor cells and healthy cells. The "coincidences" continue. Rick Smalley was a Nobel Prize winner for the discovery of carbon nanotubes, hollow cylinders of pure carbon measuring about a billionth of a meter. Smalley just "happened" to be another cancer patient at M. D. Anderson under the care of Dr. Curley. They both agreed to work together with Smalley providing the nanotubes for Curley's research. Using the therapy on tumor-injected rats and rabbits has proven it very effective. Their work has caught the attention of numerous researchers and institutions. At the time of this writing, the M. D. Anderson Cancer Center is leading the effort. Dr. Curley is managing the project after Kanzius died in February of 2009 as a result of his cancer. Dr. Curley's primary concentration now is to use special molecules attached to the nanotubes which are programmed to target only cancer cells. The NCI, in October, 2009, granted $2.1 million to the research over a five-year period. M. D. Anderson expects clinical trials on humans to be three or four years away.

The Potential is Unlimited

I closed this chapter with the radio wave example to show how broad the spectrum of potential integrative treatment options is. Not only do we need to pursue natural nutrients, look back into ancient medicine, exploit newly discovered technology, and reconsider certain previously rejected remedies. We also need to search for the unimagined, like John Kanzius did. Radio wave and nanoparticles technology applied to cancer is intriguing, but it may prove to be invalid for humans after a few years of testing. Regardless, we must keep searching, keep experimenting, keep hoping, and keep believing. If a radio guy can discover a non-intrusive alternative therapy possibility that ignites serious research by top medical research institutions, what else could there be out there? The problem is that this is not a common story. It does not happen very often. There are many people like John Kanzius in the world who need many professionals like Dr. Steven Curley with connections to many resources like those of the M. D. Anderson Cancer Center. If enough recognized medical researchers and institutions start paying attention to the potential of natural, less invasive treatment options, I believe a cure for most types of cancers will be forthcoming.

A military strategy of concentrated frontal assault works only when the enemy is inferior. A frontal assault strategy for cancer that hasn't been able to declare victory in a half century certainly proves that the enemy is not inferior. In fact, this enemy has resisted almost all conventional tactics and progressive weapons used against it. The strategy must change to include new tactics that focus more on the enemy's weaknesses. Every enemy has weaknesses. We must find ways to penetrate its vulnerable flanks. We must learn how it thinks, how to intercept its support, how to cut off its supply lines, where to strike with precision for maximum damage, how to disrupt, disorganize, and demoralize its forces, and how to break its codes to discover its plans. The new strategy must also give our own forces maximum advantage through protective armor, better detecting systems, and faster, more flexible maneuvering.

Our failing cancer war strategy is illustrated in the biblical account of David and Goliath. The Israelites and the Philistines had been battling for many days with Israel's very existence at stake. With both sides heavily armored and armed, the stalemate war came down to one Philistine who could tip the scale in his nation's favor. A nine-foot tall "giant" named Goliath challenged the Israelites to a one-on-one fight, winner take all. The Israelites could find no one among their ranks who could possibly prevail against this giant with impenetrable armor, formidable weapons, and intimidating size. Then a young Israelite shepherd boy, unknown, not even a part of the army, stepped forward. He was probably the least likely giant challenger in all of Israel from the perspectives of seasoned combatants on both sides. David approached the giant with no armor, no sword— just a small stone in a slingshot. That stone, however, entered the only tiny opening in the giant's armor, the eye slit, sank deeply into his forehead, and killed him instantly. David hit the only unprotected square inch of the giant's body and the only part of his body that assured the kill. This was totally unconventional warfare conducted by a totally unknown and unproven combatant.

The promising unconventional solutions presented in this chapter are just a few of many that vary in their position in the waiting line of good scientific evaluation. Any and all must be scientifically scrutinized to the acceptance standards of the medical community. You may have noticed that information presented on most of the examples in this chapter included the comment that more research and testing were needed. We don't need to be doing <u>more</u> research as much as we need to be doing the <u>right</u> research. Good science is not just improving on past practices. Good science is excluding nothing from the realm of possibilities. The new strategy for the war on cancer must ensure that new and peripheral methods and medicines compete in the laboratories of our finest academic and scientific institutions.

CHAPTER 7

THE PIONEERS OF COMPLEMENTARY AND ALTERNATIVE MEDICINE (CAM) CANCER TREATMENT

Thousands of years before the beginning of medical science as it is defined today, alternative medicine as it is defined today was, in fact, what medical practitioners practiced. What did our ancient ancestors do for those who were sick? They depended on natural botanicals and minerals for medicines.

The first use of plants as healing agents were found illustrated in the cave paintings discovered in the <u>Lascaux</u> caves in France. Those crude drawings have been carbon dated between 13,000 and 25,000 BC. Throughout the history of mankind, self-appointed or trained medical craftsmen have used the resources of plant and animal life to cure the infirmed. Although materials and techniques differed from culture to culture, commonalities can be observed in anthropological studies of various populations.

About 4,000 years ago, alchemy began to surface as a complement to the use of herbal remedies in the field of healing. Alchemy encompassed numerous philosophical traditions spanning the three continents of Asia, Africa, and Europe. It was originally the study of the transformation of one type of substance, usually metal, into another. Making gold from a common metal was the dream. Webster defines alchemy as the process of transforming something common into something precious.

Plant alchemy, or "spagyric," was an outgrowth of the quest for mineral transmutations. For centuries, scholars sought to find elixir remedies resulting from their "experiments" with the earthen and organic elements. Bi-products of this effort were compounds taken internally or applied externally as medications. Biblical references to anointing the infirmed with oils had both a spiritual and physical connotation as mineral oils conveyed healing properties to the body. Those bearing the title of alchemist were the pharmacists of that era.

Until the 16th century, alchemy was the centerpiece of scientific endeavor, particularly in Europe. Isaac Newton occupied himself much more in the study of alchemy than of physics for which he is remembered. Man's infatuation with this multi-faceted pursuit began to decline in the 1700's with the birth of chemistry, a more precise and reliable framework for matter transmutations. The 19th century ushered in a medicine revolution with advances in chemistry and laboratory techniques and equipment. Antiquated theories regarding infectious disease were replaced with breakthroughs in bacteriology. Louis Pasteur's linkage of microorganisms with disease brought yet another revolution in the analysis and curing of diseases. Unprecedented leaps in medical science continued into the 20th century when the application of new scientific methodology began to produce amazing developments in pharmacology and surgery.

The 20th century concurrently witnessed a shift from a master-apprentice paradigm of teaching clinical medicine to a more universal system of medical schools. The vaccinations against deadly diseases, the triumphs over tuberculosis and polio, and the development of antibiotics have revolutionized the health care of the last few generations. These and numerous others phenomenal medical successes have, in many ways, caused an institutional atmosphere of invulnerability. University medical centers, especially in America, teach that the successes of the past century form the foundation from which to build a limitless model for post-modern medicine. Although that approach has promise for many aspects of health care, cancer has not shown to be appreciably affected by what has worked in the recent past.

The medical establishment of the Western World has carried the relatively unsuccessful response to cancer across the threshold of the 21st century. The institutionalized medical education system continues to graduate doctors and technicians who have been taught that the surgical and chemical drug breakthroughs of the past century have universal application to all diseases. In general, their focus is on the disease rather than the person. It is on the symptom rather than the cause. It is on killing the erring organism rather than eradicating the organism's support. It is on infusing artificial compounds to weaken the opposition rather than strengthening the body's natural defenses. Again, this approach may be acceptable for many physical issues, but it has not been effective enough for cancer. Yet, in America and most industrialized nations, it remains the only practical choice for cancer patients.

Throughout the polarization of most medical professionals around institutionalized allopathy, a minority contingent has continued to combine the historical fundamentals with futuristic discoveries. These pioneers of complementary and alternative practices seek to rise above the status quo of the medical and pharmaceutical establishment. Like the alchemists, they maintain a vision of transforming something common into something precious.

CAM Pioneers

When most people think of pioneers in the medical field, they think of people like Alexander Fleming who introduced penicillin or Jonas Salk, discoverer of the polio vaccine, or Michael DeBakey, the patriarch of cardiovascular surgery. Any list of pioneering medical institutions would probably include the Mayo Clinic, Johns Hopkins Medical System, Memorial Sloan-Kettering Cancer Center, and M. D. Anderson Cancer Center. These names should certainly be counted among the headliners of medical advances for which we all owe a tremendous debt of gratitude. However, there are other names and institutions that have, for years, been dedicated to the furthering of medical science, but their names are virtually unrecognized.

There are highly professional, exceedingly educated, and successfully tested medical practitioners among us today who have melded the legacy of their forefathers' practices with the science of modern medicine. Most of these professionals have degrees from some of the most revered medical schools. They have initially practiced conventional medicine and research within the established system. However, their respect for the time-proven concepts and principles of healing arts over the centuries combined with their application of modern scientific medicine are believed to be not only compatible, but very advantageous, to their patients. The problem is that institutional medicine in America is very reluctant to allow the two realms to integrate for the best results. The pressures of the American Medical Association (AMA), the pharmaceutical industry, and the government often force these practitioners to the periphery of accepted practice. They are left to either acquiesce to restricted practice, accept limitations on their research, or even to move outside of our borders.

I personally interviewed a couple of these key professionals in CAM research and practice. These practitioners span a broad spectrum of emphases and philosophies. They are the early adopters and present day protagonists for what is the hope for the war on cancer.

Drs. Ernesto Contreras, Sr. and Francisco Contreras

Dr. Ernesto Contreras, Sr., a citizen of Mexico, received his post graduate training in 1939 at Harvard Children's Hospital in Boston, part of Harvard University. Returning to Mexico, he became the professor of histology and pathology at the Mexican Army Medical School. For a few years, he divided his practice between Tijuana, Mexico, and San Diego. Mercy Hospital in San Diego offered him a full-time position, but he declined in favor of serving in his own country. Most likely, a factor in that decision was his experience with the increasingly restrictive pressures placed on doctors in America to limit their practices to conventional standards. In the early 1960's, when chemotherapy and radiation became the only therapies considered by doctors who had been schooled solely in those procedures, Dr. Contreras began receiving more and more patients crossing the border for the hope that was not being given by their own country's doctors.

One such patient was Cecile Hoffman. Cecile had suffered grueling rounds of chemotherapy and had been told by her oncologist that there was no hope for her survival. She had read about a new cancer drug available in Canada called laetrile. After traveling to Canada to obtain the drug, she asked Dr. Contreras to oversee her use of it. Since laetrile had not been accepted by the U.S. Food and Drug Administration, it was not legal in her own country. As the treatments progressed, Cecile became stronger and showed signs of cancer reduction. Within months, Cecile Hoffman's cancer had disappeared. Given the death sentence under conventional treatment, here was another example of healing a cancer patient with the use of a natural substance (laetrile has been categorized as a vitamin and given the name, vitamin B_{17}). As mentioned in Chapter 6, it is found in the pits of certain fruits, principally the apricot, and has been subjected to much criticism.

Word of mouth spread as cancer patients flooded the small Tijuana office for treatment of various cancers. Embracing his vision of treating the whole person, Dr. Contreras embarked on a life-long mission to improve the treatment of catastrophic diseases through attention to the physical, emotional, and spiritual care of his patients. He committed himself to the use of any means that proved to be both effective and harmless to those who were suffering. No therapy was to be off-limits as long as it was potentially successful and qualified by his two absolutes: (1) do no harm and (2) treat the patient as yourself. That vision led to the establishment of what is now the Oasis of Hope Hospital on the Pacific coast of Tijuana, Mexico.

Today, the Oasis of Hope Hospital continues to be guided by the vision and philosophy of Dr. Contreras. It is now under the direction of his son, Dr. Francisco Contreras. After graduation from medical schools in Mexico and California, the younger Contreras completed his surgical oncology studies at Vienna, Austria. He has developed the Oasis of Hope into a full service, state of the art hospital with 120 private rooms. Since it was founded by his father in 1963, the hospital has been the venue of treatment for over 100,000 patients. Dr. Contreras now oversees the care of about 400 cancer patients annually. Typically, patients from over a dozen nations at any given week are having nutritional, organic, and customized meals together. They are engaging in group social activities, enjoying mutual worship and devotional opportunities, and encouraging each other.

The majority of patients arriving at the Oasis of Hope have Stage Four cancer—cancer that has metastasized, or transported itself, to other areas and organs of the body. Since this level is usually diagnosed as being terminal, people come with feelings of defeat and desperation. The worst-case patient is led to understand that their cancer may not be cured, but that it can be held in check allowing many more years of normal life. Dr. Contreras' objective is to make a cancer victim a cancer victor by controlling the disease to the category of a chronic condition much like diabetes.

Most visits to Oasis of Hope are about three weeks is length. After reviewing past medical records and conducting several comparative tests, the patient is prescribed a protocol of treatments personally designed for his or her particular needs. These may include laetrile drips, juicing, colonic irrigation, detoxification, vitamin therapy, oxygenation, and hydrotherapy. Surgery and chemotherapy are used sparingly and when there is a certainty of positive results. Integrated with the treatment is substantial education and training in nutrition (essentially vegetarian), lifestyle, and medications. Prescribed medications are taken home by the patient to be self-administered after the residential stay. An open ended period of consultation and follow-up visits is offered as needed.

Patients are encouraged to bring their spouse or other accompanying partner for the treatment. The partner attends all of the educational session and is a motivator for the patient. He or she stays in the same room with the patient and learns how to care for the patient after the treatment visit.

Dr. Francisco Contreras is a widely known and respected oncologist. He has become a renowned spokesperson for the combining of conventional and CAM therapies including emotional and spiritual support. He has written ten books including, *The Coming Cancer Cure, The Hope of Living Cancer Free,* and *Dismantling Cancer*. He hosts or is the keynote speaker of numerous medical conferences and conventions each year. He has been a prolific author of many articles in medical journals and magazines. I first met Dr. Contreras when Connie was a patient at Oasis of Hope in 2001 after her conventional treatment in the U.S. offered no further hope. The research for this book afforded me the opportunity to travel again to Mexico and interview Dr. Contreras in his hospital office.

My visit with him brought back both happy and sad memories. Seven years earlier, I had arrived at the mauve-colored, multi-level facility with Connie after running out of options. I had found the hospital web site after searching almost frantically for some kind of next move after our devastating experience with my dear wife's metastasized, Stage Four breast cancer. Our oncologist, only after I insisted on a bottom-line appraisal of Connie's chances for survival, informed us that she had only a short time to live. The oncologist concluded that everything that could be done had been done. A few emails and phone calls later, we reserved round-trip airline tickets to San Diego. The hospital would meet us at the airport with van transportation across the border to the facility.

Now, visiting again without the stressful circumstances of the first visit, I was, nevertheless, overwhelmed with emotion. While waiting for my interview with Dr. Contreras, I wandered into the dining room where I could still visualize the faces of quickly acquired friends. It is amazing how fast strangers can bond like family when the commonality of cancer co-exists with the mutual hope of recovery. We would sit at those tables eating our vegetables and fruits while talking with patients, often from another continent, about the details of our infirmity. We would even share the graphic accounts of the day's treatments—probably more than the other couple really wanted to know. But, it was patients touching the lives of other patients in a clinical setting, something that just doesn't happen in the typical American medical environment.

I slowly walked down a hallway of the first floor that I thought I remembered correctly. About three-fourths of the way down the hallway, I paused at the closed door of the room we occupied for several days. Not much had changed. Directly across the hall were the continuous brewing pots for our green tea along with pitchers of various natural juices. I remembered standing in our doorway and greeting other patients and their partners who would come to get their prescribed drinks. Connie was usually asleep. She was constantly exhausted. All of the memories and mixed emotions were rekindled. Yet, it was a peaceful feeling as I replayed those days in my mind. To this day, I still firmly believe that we were supposed to be there. When I compare and contrast that experience with what we had experienced in the prior three years with conventional medicine, I am even more convinced than ever that victory over this dreadful disease lies more in environs like these than in the aloof settings of most cancer centers. Probably the answer is in a combination of both.

Dr. Contreras was very polite and easy to talk with, as I remembered him being. It was like visiting with an old friend. Although I had not visited with him at length before, I felt that I knew him personally through his books that I had read. He spoke with authority and passion.

I began with a very broad and open-ended question: what must we be doing first and foremost in the war against cancer? He said that we must be focused on two areas. First, prevention is our biggest weapon. He believes that much more money and effort should be directed to educating the public about how to prevent cancer. A significant percentage of public and private funding should go toward helping industry as a whole to understand the role that carcinogenic pollutants in the air, water, and food play in the proliferation of cancer. Industry needs to be given incentive to research how to operate at a profit without tainting the environment. People need to know how to more easily avoid contaminated food, air, and other matter.

Dr. Contreras feels that our second priority should be to improve both the life expectancy and quality of life for those whose cancer has progressed beyond a reasonable expectation of cure. He stressed that we need to be developing better therapies that will control the tumor from growing and spreading even when there is very little chance to eradicate the tumor. Sometimes people die from relatively small tumors in complicated, highly sensitive areas of the body. A small tumor in the heart or brain for example can be deadly. Other tumors may be much larger, but in less impacting areas and can be destroyed or controlled before they spread to other areas and the patient lives indefinitely. Only about 10 percent of all cancer patients die from primary tumors that have not metastasized to other organs. Ninety percent of cancer deaths are from metastasized tumors.

"The real difference in Oasis of Hope and many other institutions is that our target is not the tumor; our target is the patient." Dr. Contreras explained. "That has always been our major thrust. Our aim is to maintain the patient's quality of life for an indefinite period of time."

"Many people would assess the stabilizing of a tumor as a failure. We don't. If a patient comes to us having been given two or three months to live, and he is alive twenty years later with X-rays showing that the tumor still exists, he is happy, and we are happy."

He said the difference in his strategy and the strategies of most conventional practitioners is philosophical, not technical. "There is a lot of money and commitment out there, but they are looking for the wrong thing. Their aim is the tumor, and the patient is secondary. Ninety percent of the research money goes to the study of the tumor, yet only 10 percent of patients die from a primary tumor. Very little money is spent to study metastasis which is what kills the patient. Rarely will you find published studies on metastasis because it is a complex condition. At Oasis, we study the metastasized tumors and help our patients cope with them. We help keep the tumors in check—keep them stabilized. If, in that process, the tumors are reduced or eliminated—and some are—praise the Lord!"

To clarify, he emphasized, "If only 10 percent or less of women die of cancer of the breast before it metastasizes to the liver or somewhere else, why is all the money being spent on cancer of the breast and very little being spent on metastasized cancer that is the real killer?"

I can personally identify with that statement. Connie had breast cancer that was declared in remission after 18 months of chemo and radiation. Three months later, breast cancer tumors were discovered on her liver. More aggressive chemo was ordered, and surgery was performed. When I finally got a straight answer regarding what was being done, it was simply that they were trying to extend her life a few more months. Basically, no amount of sophisticated processes or procedures could significantly extend the life of a Stage Four cancer victim. And, her last months were debilitating. I am so thankful that Dr. Contreras and others outside the mainstream of medicine are pursuing this research and practice involving Stage Four of cancer.

I asked if he thought there was hope for a changed mindset in mainstream medicine.

"I think you are seeing a slight movement toward a new philosophy, although slowly. It almost has to change, because the hopes of finding a cure are vanishing despite the tremendous amount of money and knowledge being dedicated to the cause. I see a few leaders in the cancer battle beginning to think as my father thought 25 years ago, that we need to concentrate on how to help the patient survive."

I understood and agreed with what he was saying about metastasized cancer. But, I was still uncertain about alternative treatment for cancer discovered in stage one. I presented him a hypothetical scenario of being diagnosed with lung cancer. Suppose a spot was found on my lung during a routine X-ray. If there were no evidence of metastasis, would I be better off with conventional treatment or should I still come to a place like Oasis of Hope for my treatment. Would he treat me with laetrile and the complementary protocols?

He was quick to respond, "In Stage One, no. For Stage One lung cancer, cervical cancer, and several other cancers, surgery will usually bring a cure. The difference in Stage One treatment of most cancers in the U.S. and what we do here is in the area of complementary treatment. We would do the very least intrusive procedures possible. If after investigating the cancer, we felt that a combination of chemotherapy and other therapies would remove the cancer, that is what we would recommend. The down side of surgery is that it carries the greater possibility of the cancer returning. But, if surgery is the best choice, that would be our recommendation. Now what we will offer that you won't get in most American hospitals is the umbrella of protection and assurance that we do everything we can to compensate for the damage that is done to your body as a result of the treatment."

I had learned from *Dismantling Cancer* that, when Oasis of Hope had to resort to surgery or chemotherapy, they complemented the procedures with treatments that strengthened the immune system, muscles, and bones. They also provided opportunities that enhanced the patient's emotional and spiritual strength for overcoming the challenging process of healing.

Dr. Contreras came full circle back to metastasis with the comment, "Now, when it comes to Stage Four cancers, we have here a much better chance of your surviving over five years than does, for instance, M. D. Anderson [Cancer Center in Houston, Texas]. We address many more issues associated with Stage Four."

I mentioned a chart in *Dismantling Cancer* (Table 7-1) that was striking in the comparison of survival rates between Oasis of Hope patients and those of conventional treatment facilities.

Table 7-1 Survival Rates for Stage IV Cancers

Type of Cancer: Distant[a]	Number of Patients	5 yr. Survival Rate %	
		Oasis	Conventional[b]
Lung Cancer	200	30	3
Breast Cancer	130	39	23
Colon Cancer	150	30	9
Prostate Cancer	600	86	34

a. Distant: A malignant cancer that has spread to parts of the body remote from the primary tumor either by direct extension or by discontinuous metastasis to distant organs, tissues, or via the lymphatic system to distant lymph nodes.
b. Source: American Cancer Society. Cancer Facts & Figures 2003.

I noted that Stage Four patients treated at Oasis had from a 70% to a 900% increase in the five year survival rate over patients with conventional treatment. That means, for instance, a patient diagnosed with metastasized lung cancer and getting treatment in America has almost no chance of being alive five years later. But, almost one in six such patients getting CAM treatments in Oasis will live at least five years and maybe longer—maybe a normal life expectancy.

I asked Dr. Contreras if there were statistics on Stage Four cancer survival beyond five years.

"The reason it is standard to stop at five years is research cost. However, statistically speaking, the chances of you living out your life after five years are quite good. In the case of cancer of the breast, research is often done to ten years, because the chances of breast cancer recurring is much greater than for other types of cancer."

I wanted to clarify that the research cost he was referring to was the expenses of collecting and analyzing the data.

"Yes, the cost of collecting data and studying that data from every angle is terribly expensive. People in the States have a lot of money for research, but for us, particularly in the alternative treatment care, even a five year study challenges our budget. And we have no help from anyone or anywhere."

I asked why he didn't have help. Why wouldn't private donors and, in his case, the Mexican Government fund some research that could scientifically prove the anecdotal conclusions of so many patients.

"The government of Mexico and the big donors in Mexico do not consider cancer research to be as important as many other problems such as poverty. I do not expect much interest in funding our research until other needs considered a higher priority are resolved. It is not that there is no interest in our work; it is just that other unfunded areas are so overwhelming."

Since America is a giving country, and billions of dollars are going from philanthropists' pockets into conventional cancer research, I suggested a scenario where Americans might be convinced to support CAM cancer research outside the country. By his quick response, Dr. Contreras had obviously entertained that suggestion before.

"I could give you a receipt for your donation, but your country would not accept it as a tax deductible donation. You cannot give money to even a non-profit organization outside your borders and file it on your taxes."

The answer, of course, is to conduct extensive research into CAM and integrative treatment within the borders of the United States. I truly believe the interest is there at the grass roots level, but it will take a lot of intense effort to move the mainstream medical and pharmaceutical establishments as well as the government into that realm.

In *Dismantling Cancer*, Dr. Contreras writes that there is much research lying dormant on the shelves of medical libraries that validates unconventional options to cancer treatment. I requested his elaboration on that. Is there indisputable evidence of solid research that is not getting anyone's attention?

"Let me give you just one of many examples. Look up the work of Dr. Mark Levine, the top researcher of the U.S. government's National Institutes of Health. He revived the whole issue of Vitamin C, proving it worthy to use with cancer patients. He is frustrated because few medical professionals want to consider it. It is being debated throughout the medical community, but Levine's research proves that Vitamin C in high doses strengthens the immune system for battling cancer cells with no harmful side effects."

We covered the Levine research in Chapter 5, but as a quick review, his studies indicate that Vitamin C could possibly be a major tumor fighter with little or no side effects. Unfortunately, he has found it difficult to convince other researchers to partner with him on conclusive studies.

Dr. Contreras' remarks about convincing research not being accepted by conventional treatment advocates gave me a segue to raise the issue of laetrile. As I anticipated, he is always ready to assume the role of laetrile's spokesperson.

"The only study ever published on the use of laetrile was sponsored by the National Cancer Institute and conducted at the Mayo Clinic along with three other prominent oncology centers in the U.S. The resulting article in *The New England Journal of Medicine (NEJM)* by researcher, Dr. Charles Moertel, concluded that not one of 178 patients accepted in the study was cured or even stabilized by laetrile. The study was completely biased. There was no control group, and not one researcher had any experience with laetrile. Normally, the NEJM will not publish anything without it being peer reviewed. I know almost every laetrile expert in the world, and not one of us was asked to review the study. What's more, even if the study was done correctly and the results were bad for laetrile, just one study proves nothing. All pharmaceuticals have been tested numerous times, often with mixed results, until enough tests become convincing."

I asked about a story in his book where his laetrile presentation at an oncology conference raised the ire of a colleague. Dr. Contreras smiled and shook his head.

"He was furious because I still advocated the use of laetrile in spite of the fact that Dr. Moertel had "proven" its danger and ineffectiveness. I asked him, 'Would you stop using Taxol (a chemotherapy agent used commonly for breast cancer) if I showed you one article that said it was not effective?' He just turned around and left. We both knew that there were studies indicating the ineffectiveness and high toxicity of Taxol, yet most oncologists prescribe it."

This story is illustrative of the way studies and testing of natural and non-pharmacological options to cancer therapy are often skewed to discount their validity. Medical research seldom provides a level playing field friendly to players from both conventional and unconventional medicine.

Dr. Contreras continued, "Now, I don't believe there is a government or industrial conspiracy to prohibit the validation of unconventional medicines and methods. It is just that the system is designed to promote the conventional and traditional. It's just like any other business. You have to have an incentive to pursue new possibilities. There is no incentive for the businesses of medicine to prove clinically that natural therapies work. There are only disincentives for that. It takes a lot of money to prove the effectiveness and safety of a new medicine, and they will never make it back if the new medicine is a natural compound that is widely available and cheap to obtain. They only pay for their research if they develop the product, keep it scarce, control its distribution, and sell it at an exorbitant price."

He brought up the potential of curcumin, the ginger-like root that I wrote about in Chapter 5 as having anti-cancer properties.

"It's interesting what is happening at M. D. Anderson [Cancer Center] with curcumin. It shows great promise in their studies, but I am convinced it is not going to be used, because there is no incentive to develop it. I don't blame the scientists. The scientists are doing what they can, but the medical and pharmaceutical industries, looking at profit and loss won't invest the money in natural therapies that they can't make a return on. When it can take an investment of billions of dollars from concept to market for most prescription drugs, who wants to test, develop, and market a remedy that you can grow in your back yard? Why would a drug company spend billions of dollars to find that an anti-cancer compound is safe and effective, when it's one they know I could make here in my hospital? "

My years of frustration regarding this subject were being shared by this icon of integrative cancer treatment. I wanted to know what he thought the answer was. I suppose I led with what I wanted to hear as I asked whether a grass roots movement from the general public, like the strategy in this book, would be successful.

"Yes, I believe it could happen. Ultimately, the federal government must legislate away many of the constraints placed on researchers, medical universities, and pharmaceutical firms. The government must also be willing to direct adequate research funding to integrative treatment research. Tax incentives and financial assistance for alternative treatment research would at least reduce some of the burden of high-dollar research and production of new complementary treatment medicines. The government must permit physicians the freedom to support the patients' rejection of exclusively conventional treatment and selection of integrative treatment. Right now in America, both you and your doctor could go to jail for choosing some forms of CAM treatments. The government works for the people, and with enough pressure, they will act on the people's behalf. Someone with the brains and economic savvy to figure all this out has to come up with a formula for making it work. I'm a doctor. I see the problem every day, but I don't have the answer."

It was a great interview. What a wise, passionate, and compassionate man. As I rode to the airport, my head buzzed with thoughts and ideas. The problem had been organized and structured in my mind perhaps better than ever before. But I kept dwelling on his last six words, "....but, I don't have the answer."

Much of the hour-long drive to the border brought me within close proximity to the seemingly endless metal fence that separated Mexico and America. I contemplated how that fence defined much more than who could be on what side of it. In general, it separated wealth from poverty, technology from manual labor, and international power from virtual isolationism. Ironically, however, when it comes to treating chronic health problems, it seems to separate a myopic view of the traditional from an open acceptance of the possible.

Dr. Myron Wentz

On the beautiful and tranquil beach of Rosarito, Mexico, on the Baja Peninsula sits the lavish Strauss mansion formally owned by the descendents of Levi Strauss (yes, the patriarch of the blue jeans empire). Next to it, and connected by a breezeway, stands a ten-floor hospital known as Sanoviv. Sanoviv, meaning "healthy life," was designed and staffed to provide a healing environment for the entire person—mind, body, and spirit. The founder of this unique medical center is Myron Wentz, Ph.D.

Dr. Wentz is an internationally acclaimed microbiologist, immunologist, and pioneer in the development of human cell culture technology and infectious disease diagnoses. After earning his master's degree in microbiology from the University of North Dakota, he graduated from the University of Utah with a doctorate in microbiology and immunology. Launching Gull Laboratories in 1974, he developed many original diagnostic tests for viral and other infectious diseases. Through his extensive research, he developed a passion for applying natural curatives to diseases, especially the chronic degenerative diseases. Based on decades of nutritional research in cell culture, he founded USANA Health Sciences in 1992, a manufacturer of nutritional supplements and health products.

His combined medical and business interests led to his purchase of the Strauss mansion and building of the hospital, together a fully accredited integrative medical center. There, he could research and implement new and promising methodologies and medications that would not be possible under the constraints of his homeland of America. His vision was to offer a first class experience whether patients were healthy and wanted to be healthier or were seeking treatment for a specific, maybe life-threatening, disease.

Cancer sufferers arriving at Sanoviv receive a thorough health assessment to identify the extent and the cause of the disease. This includes functional, biochemical, physical, psychological and bioenergetics testing.   The treatment program is then customized to employ all necessary natural medicine, methods and techniques to stop the disease process and to maximize immunological involvement and responsiveness.

This physical care is liberally supplemented with attention to the mind and soul. I visited Sanoviv, and found it to be a unique and intriguing operation. The first impression is awe inspiring. The landscaping, therapy pools, contemporary furnishings, and ocean views through endless glass windows provide a pampered atmosphere designed specifically for those being cared for.   The comfortable patient rooms, unlike typical hospital rooms, are in a luxurious setting. The cost of the stay and care is reasonable relative to the amenities.

Sanoviv attends to much more than just the physical needs. Professional nutritionists educate the patient in proper nutrition and food preparation tailored to ones personal metabolism and particular health needs. Only highly nutritious and organic foods are served. Sanoviv prides itself in having the most advanced detoxification capabilities to rid the body environmental toxics. Psychologists work with each individual to deal with negative emotions and memories that surface during whole body detoxification. Spiritual counselors help patients gain healing advantage through their own journey of faith. The majority of Sanoviv's physicians, dentists, chiropractors, nutritionists and psychologist are certified in functional medicine by the Institute of Functional Medicine headquartered in the United States. From the physicians to the therapists to the biological dentists, the objective is to treat the whole person, not just the cancer.

Sanoviv offers many options under one roof, all of which are leading edge applications of the latest in treatments. They do not use therapies that damage and weaken the overall body. Instead the body's environment is influenced to be adverse to and reject malignancy. Body alkalization, oxygenation and hyperthermia therapies are used most commonly with bioenergetics, immune enhancement, and biological response modifiers as an integral part of most therapy regimens. In addition anticancer phytochemicals and orthomolecular nutrition play key roles in Sanoviv's protocols.

Cancer cells require an acidic environment to grow. An alkalinizing diet helps greatly to restore proper pH to the body. Oxygen is toxic to cancer cells. Sanoviv has a very impressive variety of ways to flood the body's cells with oxygen including hyperbaric oxygenation and extracorporeal ozonation. Cancer cells are more sensitive to heat than normal cells. Whole body hyperthermia therapy elevates body temperature to carefully controlled levels. Regional hyperthermia is also used effectively.

Immunotherapy and enzyme therapy have been shown to have powerful anticancer benefits and are routinely used in most therapy programs. Immunotherapy not only restores immune system function but is used to specifically stimulate Natural Killer cells, Tumor Necrosis Factor, and T cells to recognize and eliminate cancer cells. Enzyme therapy along with nutrition, toxicology, and hydrotherapy support detoxification which is core to Sanoviv.

Natural medicines and phytochemicals are used to inhibit angiogenesis (formations of new blood vessels) as well as to inhibit certain growth factors (stimulators of cell proliferation). Some phytochemicals actually promote transformation of malignant cells back into normal cells. Other phytochemicals inhibit tumor growth directly. One of the important objectives of natural medicines and therapies at Sanoviv according to Dr. Wentz is to promote p53 expression to initiate apoptosis of cancer cells (cell suicide). The protein, p53, is a natural tumor suppressor produced by the body.

Sanoviv practices "functional nutrition," an emerging new system of clinical assessment and intervention that takes conventional nutrition to the next level by understanding the root causes and imbalances in cellular function that result from improper or inadequate diet. Sanoviv's intravenous administration of certain nutrients focuses primarily on antioxidant protection from carcinogens, avoidance of carcinogens directly, and support of the immune system.

Dr. Danielle Aguiniga, Sanoviv's Chief of Staff commented, "We are also seeing great potential with biological therapies involving the use of selected white blood cells to fight cancer. The National Polytechnic Institute (IPN) in Mexico has discovered that certain white blood cell factors from a cancer survivor are especially effective when introduced into the blood system of a patient with a similar cancer. We are sending biopsy tissues from some of our patients to IPN which makes laboratory matches to white blood cells of donors who have battled the same type of cancer. This process is still rather new, but the initial results are very promising. The best results seem to be with kidney, lymphoma, and breast cancers."

Understanding that much of the leading edge therapy at Sanoviv was proving to be effective, I was still not sure what it all meant for survivability of the patient. Dr. Aguiniga explained.

"Since most of our patients are with us for only a few weeks, one of our challenges is follow-up. We try to establish a coordinated effort with the patient's doctor after our treatment to include regular dialog regarding medicines and tests. We also request questionnaire responses from the patient. Post-treatment data are kept by a special department within our organization. We encourage our patients to return to Sanoviv quarterly or semiannually for follow-up checkups."

Sanoviv is certainly a fascinating and impressive cancer treatment institution. I believe its practitioners hold a lot of hope for the war on cancer. Developing treatment options at a pace that seems foreign (no pun intended) to the American medical community, they surge ahead while we often languish in the mire of redundant testing and bureaucratic processes. Some of what is being practiced in Sanoviv and other Mexican institutions is illegal north of the border. Its illegality is not necessarily because the treatment is thought not to work; it is often because of restrictions from the complex and lengthy approval process under which the United States medical system chooses to operate. Unless and until institutionalized medicine, the pharmaceutical industry, and the federal government adopt a more permissive approach to cancer research and treatment, U. S. citizens will continue to be deprived of potential breakthroughs that could save or extend lives.

CAM Is Not Synonymous with Quackery

It is apparent from the medical professionals and facilities highlighted in this chapter that CAM, for the most part, is a highly legitimate field. The complementary part of it is scientifically proven and should be practiced more. The alternative part of it that has not been tested should be prioritized and the most promising practices expedited in clinical trials. It holds great promise for victory over a myriad of diseases, including cancer. There are enough examples of trustworthy achievers like those in this chapter to write a book of Who's Who in CAM. Maybe I will do that someday. Of course, there have been too many quack doctors, worthless potions, and phony clinics in the recent history of alternative medicine. We must be extremely cautious as we move ahead in the progress of CAM, complementary cancer therapy in particular, to restore public confidence in the movement. We must be especially selective in who and what are placed on the front lines in the battle against cancer. The voices of integrative oncology must be legitimate and of utmost integrity. Its ambassadors have to earn the confidence and respect of stakeholders throughout the entire field of medicine. Like emissaries in foreign countries, integrative oncologists must work within the often skeptical culture to realize their objectives. Victory in the war on cancer will require the best commanders to use the latest technology in deploying unconventional forces in combination with conventional forces.

CHAPTER 8

THE PRACTITIONERS OF
INTEGRATIVE ONCOLOGY

Let's review some terms briefly. We have just highlighted complementary and alternative medicine (CAM) cancer treatment pioneers. CAM includes both complementary medicine that is "added to" conventional treatment as well as alternative medicine that is used "instead of" conventional treatment. Integrative medicine is practiced by providers who choose to use complementary medicine to enhance the efficacy and lessen the negative impact of conventional medicine. Integrative practitioners focus on the whole person in treating diseases. They usually disregard alternative medicine unless or until it is scientifically proven in clinical trials. For instance, integrative oncologists practice natural, non-toxic complementary therapies to enhance the conventional therapies. The term *CAM* seems to be giving way to the term *integrative medicine* as the science of unconventional medicine matures. Integrative medicine involves the treating of the whole person rather than just the disease. The integrative oncologists and researchers practicing today are gaining a strong voice in the medical community, but are nevertheless a small minority among their conventional peers. There are many dedicated professionals in the research and practice of integrative oncology who would be worthy of recognizing, but I will showcase only a couple as very worthy representatives of the field.

Dr. Susan Folkman

At the time of this interview, Susan Folkman, Ph.D, was the founding Director of the Osher Center for Integrative Medicine and the Osher Foundation's Distinguished Professor of Integrative Medicine at University of California, San Francisco (UCSF). She recently retired earning the title of Professor Emeritus from UCSF. Dr. Folkman continues to serve on the NIH/NCCAM National Advisory Council. For over thirty years, she has been a prominent and respected leader in medical research. She was a member of the Institute of Medicine panel on CAM use in the US and is past chair (2005 – 2007) of the Consortium of Academic Health Centers for Integrative Medicine (CAHCIM)

The Osher Center for Integrative Medicine at UCSF, which Dr. Folkman directed, is taking the lead in researching complementary therapies and educating its doctors in advising their patients who seek out these therapies. The Center is named for Bernard Osher, creator of the Bernard Osher Foundation. This organization's board is now chaired by Mr. Osher's wife, Barbro Osher. Numerous integrative medicine programs and institutions benefit from the Osher Foundation's generous grants. Osher Centers are also located at Harvard Medical School and Brigham and Women's Hospital in Boston and at the Karolinska Institute in Stockholm, Sweden.

The CAHCIM, which Dr. Folkman formerly chaired, includes 44 highly esteemed academic medical centers. These medical schools are partnering in collaborative efforts to transform medicine and healthcare through rigorous scientific studies that integrate complementary and conventional medicine. Their studies explore new models of clinical care that acknowledge the intrinsic nature of healing and the diversity of therapeutic systems. Member institutions include the University of California at Irvine, Los Angeles, and San Francisco; Yale University; Johns Hopkins University; Harvard Medical School; Mayo Clinic; Columbia University; Duke University; and the University of North Carolina to name just a few.

I visited with Dr. Folkman in her UCSF office and discussed with her the outlook for CAM or integrative medicine as it relates to cancer treatment. Early in our discussion, it became apparent that she didn't totally share my assessment that there has been too little progress in conventional cancer treatment. She pointed out that survival rates have increased markedly in several types of cancer and noted leukemia and Hodgkin's as prime examples. She attributed these and other successes to conventional medicine. Early stage breast cancer, she reminded, is now survived routinely thanks to medical and pharmaceutical research and development. Her years deeply involved in medical science have given her an understanding and appreciation of how long it takes to go from theory to practice in the battle against cancer. Dr. Folkman sees integrative medicine's role as helping people sustain themselves during conventional treatment. It is important in altering people's lifestyle to prevent cancers instigated by certain behaviors.

During the first several minutes of the interview, I began wondering how and why Dr. Folkman was so prominent in the arena of CAM and integrative medicine research. She seemed to be coming across as a traditionalist in defense of conventional treatment. Then came the "however" as she emphasized that cures for many cancers are going to come from diverse areas of research and study. She said that everything should be on the table. Conventional medicine should continue to be pursued aggressively while intently looking for solutions from alternative healing systems that may be dormant outside of our awareness.

Dr. Folkman does not believe that "a cure for cancer" will come from any scientific source, whether conventional or alternative. She pointed out that cancer is ubiquitous. It has too many sources and comes in too many forms. If we find something that proves successful against one type of cancer, it may not be effective against other types. There may be a form of cancer that is responsive to a particular extract or botanical, and we need to pursue such potential. But, we should not concentrate solely on alternative possibilities. Her position is that, although CAM will not likely be an all-encompassing cure for cancer, it will improve the quality and length of life for those with cancer. CAM is incredibly important to the cancer patient's ability to survive and thrive with the disease. As we progressively realize the benefits of years and billions of dollars of conventional research, we need to understand that this research is not focused on the individual, but rather on the disease. Empowering the patient in mind, body, and spirit to combat the cancer is the crucial role of CAM.

This led me to the bottom-line question, "Why do you think there will never be an actual cure for cancer?"

Her reply was that thinking about a cure for cancer was like thinking about a cure for life itself. Life is too diverse, and cancer is too diverse, for a single answer. Certain cancers may be completely cured through advances in genetic research, stem cell applications, and certain molecular and biological discoveries. Breakthroughs are happening now and will continue to happen. We will never be able to prescribe a pill to all cancer patients and heal them. The complex array of cancers attacking the complex array of organs and systems will continue to require tremendous time and effort to eradicate. Conventional medicine and CAM are completely legitimate and are both worthy of science, but neither provides the singular answer.

Understanding Dr. Folkman's position, I asked whether she agreed that, on balance, there needed to be more emphasis on complementary medicine, particularly as it applies to integrative oncology.

The single-word preface to her answer was "absolutely." She clarified, "There is tremendous potential in complementary medicine to prevent disease, to treat disease, and to ensure the health and well-being of all people, particularly those facing cancer. So many diseases, especially cancer, are contracted or worsened by stress—physical, mental, and emotional. Much of what is going on in CAM has to do with helping the patient develop strength in body, mind, and spirit. The healing process depends on the strength within as well as the infusion of external agents. This vital aspect of healing is not the purview of conventional medicine. It is not even within the scope of psychological or behavioral practice. So, one would say it is not yet in the mainstream of care for chronic diseases. There are, therefore, huge contributions yet to be made by integrative medicine. Whether CAM will ultimately bring a significant increase in cancer survival rates is yet to be determined. But, there is no question that it holds the key to quality of life and life extension for those who are living with cancer. We certainly need to be pursuing the research and practice of CAM with much higher priority."

Dr. Folkman inserted that, in the interest of full disclosure, she wanted me to know that her brother-in-law, Dr. Judah Folkman, had conducted some very revealing and positive research into anti-angiogenesis cancer therapy. She supports his findings and expects them to be crucial in future developments of alternative therapy. You learned about his findings in Chapter 6.

I brought up the questionable research and clinical trial processes by which conventional medicine has rejected so many unconventional medicine proposals. Many CAM practitioners consider tests of numerous such cancer treatments within conventional medicine institutions to have been biased if not sabotaged in order to disprove the treatments.

Short of affirming my implication of institutional bias, Dr. Folkman agreed that every promising option deserves a fair scientific evaluation. Anytime there is a plausible explanation as to why a previous trial may have failed, it should be reintroduced. If there is reasonable evidence that something should work, then it should be open game for more testing. Conventional research routinely has both false negatives and false positives that have to be resolved through new tests. New drugs are often found initially to be ineffective, but when tested repeatedly in different doses or varying applications, their effectiveness is validated. A good example is Thalidomide developed and tested effective to reduce nausea during pregnancy. It helped the nausea, but caused birth defects in babies. The drug was banned for years. Later research found Thalidomide to be helpful in cancer treatment with no appreciable side effects. It is currently being used successfully, and on-going research shows potential for expanded advantage. Therefore, medical researchers should never reject any treatment option until it has been thoroughly tested under widely varied conditions. We could be rejecting the very thing we are looking for.

Dr. Folkman offered a very interesting comparison that is often overlooked in the medical community. Thousands of drugs for specific cancers are being tested constantly. Let us assume that 100 of these make the cut for phase I trials. Maybe only two will reach credibility for phase II. The public, even most medical and pharmaceutical professionals, will never hear of the thousands of original contender drugs that failed. On the other hand, there are thousands of botanicals, procedures, diets, and natural compounds that have been used by alternative medicine proponents for years—perhaps centuries—and probably only a very few really work. Conventional medicine proponents will look at the thousands of alternative failures as evidence that alternative medicine does not work. They neglect to give a fair and impartial assessment of the few that do work. They go to great lengths to find the conventional drugs that work, but ignore the alternative means that might have similar benefits.

I asked for her perspective on how we can convince the conventional medicine community to urgently look beyond their world even further toward promising, but unproven, concepts.

She used the analogy of our nation's long and difficult move toward the use of automobile seat belts. It will take substantial time and significant influence from a multitude of sources. She believes this book will be one such source. As more cancer patients opt for integrative treatment, they will see the good in it and will spread the word. As more people desire a more integrative approach to treatment, more doctors will seek to learn more about it. Medical schools will teach more CAM due to demand from the students and from research that proves it viable. It will take many voices to make this happen.

As our session came to a close, Dr. Folkman made a statement that I want to quote verbatim. It was a succinct, but poignant summation of her professional philosophy.

"I come from the world where science is well respected and well regarded. We are integrating medicine within that context. That is the future, I think. I don't think we should set ourselves up as 'us versus them'. It should be 'us in addition to them'. We don't take the place of conventional medicine; we add to conventional medicine. There may be some cases where conventional medicine doesn't work at all, and maybe we have something that can help. Our work in integrative oncology having to do with diet and nutrition might be the only resort where all other treatment has failed. It may not cure the person, but may make the person feel better during this period. Who knows? It might have a beneficial healing effect. This is a different stance than some of the more militant CAM supporters will take. Some will say that conventional medicine is not useful, and that we should be embracing only these alternative healing traditions that people have been using for thousands of years. I am not in that camp. I am in the camp where there is benefit in integrative medicine that can make very important contributions to the health of our society and is in addition to conventional medicine."

As noted previously, Dr. Folkman and I began the interview with somewhat differing views. However, I respect her position and agree much more than disagree with her. If complementary treatment is to get its day in the court of public opinion, it will be because dedicated researchers like her are willing to be open minded about unconventional revelations from evidenced-based scientific pursuit.

Dr. William Buchholz

In my selection of an integrative oncologist in the United States to interview, I wanted someone who was not practicing in conjunction with a prominent medical school or major cancer center. I was looking for one who represented the dedicated entrepreneur doctor that might set up an integrative practice in almost any city in the country. This person would be a model for what I hope will become the typical expectation of cancer patients across the nation. He or she would be highly experienced in both conventional and complementary therapies, but not connected to a large institution. This setting would be the norm for the new strategy for the war on cancer. My preferred profile was personified in Dr. William Buchholz.

Dr. Buchholz is the founder and sole oncologist for the Buchholz Medical Group in Mountain View, California. His interest in the holistic approach to cancer treatment began three decades ago when such practice was extremely unpopular within the medical community. His years of experience with complementary therapies are evident in the book, *Live Longer, Live Larger*, co-authored by him and his wife, Susan Buchholz, PhD. Dr. Susan Buchholz is a clinical psychologist who partners with her husband by providing psychological consultation for cancer patients. Doctors Bill and Susie, as they are affectionately called by some friends and patients, bring a unique synergy to cancer treatment that is a fresh and welcomed option for many patients.

I wanted to begin this interview on a philosophical note by asking Dr. Buchholz just why he practices integrative oncology.

"I go with what works." He replied. He further explained that, earlier in his career, he became well aware of the limits of conventional, or allopathic, medicine. Conventional medicine is concentrated almost exclusively on the disease. The body's ability to fight the disease is of little concern to those who provide treatment from a solely conventional perspective.

"I want to be 'inclusive.'" He emphasized. He asked rhetorically why anyone would not want to include every possible treatment that was not harmful and had been proven to be helpful. He has made treatment of the whole person his life calling.

Dr. Buchholz became interested in integrative medicine before he even entered medical school. He had studied psychology and philosophy in addition to pre-med and became interested in Asian philosophies.

"When I left Harvard for Stanford Medical School in 1967, there was an intense interest within some circles of medicine in innovative modalities," Dr. Buchholz noted. "My experiences convinced me that there were powerful impacts from these modalities that go beyond or at least supplement what is possible with conventional medicine. Stanford was at the educational center of these concepts and would allow me to individually explore all manner of innovative medicine." Stanford and the neighboring University of California at San Francisco have two of the most advanced medical schools in integrative medicine.

Upon his certification as an oncologist, Dr. Buchholz became closely associated with those few colleagues who were passionate about integrative oncology. He continues to be involved in Commonweal which is headed by Michael Lerner, PhD, who was quoted in Chapter 4. Commonweal is a multi-faceted organization that engages in educational, charitable, and research efforts that, in large measure, support weeklong resident programs for cancer patients. There, these patients learn about how they might benefit from various natural treatments that complement their mainstream treatments. Dr. Buchholz has consulted for Dr. Lerner and Commonweal.

I spoke of my frustration over the slow progress of integrative medicine in general and integrative oncology in particular. Dr. Buchholz sees the mainstream medical science and health care industries as suspicious of alternative medicine because it does not conform to the scientific model. Although some medical schools and medical centers have made major advancements in teaching and practicing inclusive medicine, these institutions as well as the pharmaceutical institutions as a whole still have little regard for anything beyond exclusive conventional medicine. He was also quick to admit that this conflict flows in both directions as complementary and alternative medicine advocates are often less than hospitable toward exclusively conventional practitioners.

I was curious as to how Dr. Buchholz was educated in integrative oncology when few schools prepare doctors in integrative medicine, and few hospitals train doctors in complementary cancer therapies. He countered that, although medical schools in general fall short of making integrative medicine a core curriculum, many schools are rapidly improving in this area.

"Other schools and medical centers such as Johns Hopkins, U. C. San Francisco, Harvard's Dana Farber, Sloan Kettering, and M. D. Anderson are acknowledging and applying integrative oncology in their classrooms and clinics. Granted, most courses are elective rather than required, but students who are interested in the subject certainly have access to it."

He acknowledged, however, that most integrative oncologists learn the specific complementary therapies on their own once they complete their oncology education and certification. They maintain a close-knit network with other oncologist of like interests and share findings and successes. Organizations like the Society of Integrative Oncologists (SIO) are growing rapidly as more and more oncologists see the advantages of new types of therapies.

"For me, it was an evolving process rather than a structured one as I read about new concepts, simply paid attention to patients, and applied, as appropriate, modalities that worked."

He compared the integrative oncology advancement to the hospice palliative care concept. Thirty years ago, hospice was dismissed by most medical professionals as ineffective, costly, and an interference in the traditional care of the terminally ill. However, its popularity among those who benefited from it gradually grew and was recognized by the medical community.

Dr. Buchholz recalled, "In 1977, I trained in one of the first programs for hospice. There was no formal training in the United States. We had to go to England. It was five to ten years later that hospice caught on by popular demand for more humane care for people who were dying."

He went on to say that, today, hospice is overwhelmingly accepted as the best care for those in the final weeks of their lives. Medicare and most insurance companies now cover the care. Yet, there are relatively few resources for institutional education for hospice physicians. It is a discipline of medicine that is largely learned from the experiences of others. We can all hope that integrative oncology develops and is accepted similarly. He commended this book for documenting the early stage of integrative oncology as, like hospice, a new and better way of practicing a critical genre of medicine.

Anxious to move on to Dr. Buchholz' personal practice, I asked about the source of his patients. Are most of the patients already interested in complementary therapies and choose him because of his expertise, or do most of them become interested through his advice and counsel? He answered that he, like most integrative oncologists, is a broad-based clinical practitioner. If patients come to him with little or no understanding of complementary therapies, he explains and recommends certain therapies according to their particular needs. Ultimately, the decision is theirs. If other patients have considerable knowledge of various therapy options, we discuss their personal goals for the treatment and come to an agreement on the protocol options. On occasion, a patient will refuse any conventional treatment and ask the doctor to just help him or her become as able as possible to fight and tolerate the disease. In that case, he ensures that the patient fully understands the pros and cons of his or her decision, and that he provides the best care possible.

He emphasized that the first thing an oncologist should do with a patient is to determine the patient's goals in the treatment. After sufficient advice and counsel from the doctor, the patient should always determine his or her treatment priorities. Then the doctor should do what the patient wants within professional ethics and consideration of their condition. He told me I might be surprised to learn that some patients, after being given this kind of control over their treatment, reveal that aggressively treating the cancer is not as important to them as living the rest of their days with dignity and quality of life. This is sometimes the case, particularly with victims of Stage Four cancer.

I requested some examples of what he typically prescribed in complementary therapies. He admitted a bias favorable to Chinese medicine. His penchant for the study of both ancient and modern Chinese healing practices has led him to believe that many of those practices have validity. Acupuncture has proven to not only relieve pain, but also to control symptoms such as nausea and vomiting. Chinese herbs and other medicinal plants, as a part of integrated treatment, have wide-ranging advantages for cancer patients including symptom management, immune system enhancement, and stamina boosting.

Nutritional tweaking of a patient's dietary patterns is usually accomplished by connecting him or her with a registered dietician. Dr. Buchholz has found that most patients realize the importance of eating healthy during cancer treatment to keep their body at peak capability for healing. The biggest diet problem is the loss of appetite that usually accompanies the conventional treatment. Dieticians that are specially trained in cancer patient nutrition can often advise, monitor, and assist patients in meal plans that are customized to overcome their particular treatment side effects.

Dr. Buchholz regularly prescribes certain physical therapies including massages for his patients. A massage therapist is part of his clinic staff. Also, physical conditioning regimens are recommended to keep the body's cardiovascular system primed for both enhancing the conventional therapies and reducing the side effects.

Although most of his recommended complementary therapies are referred to other professionals, Dr. Buchholz is personally and directly involved in creating a mind state with his patients that focuses on their will to live. He devotes whatever time and effort it takes to lead his patients through an introspective process that allows them to confront the disease and become determined to defeat it. He explains that cancer is a disease of cellular misinformation. DNA mutations happen all the time and sometimes get out of control. Certain lifestyle behaviors can cause this dysfunction. Some inherited proclivities cause it. The good news is that it can be altered by behavior. Conventional therapy complemented by physical-oriented therapies foster the body's attacks on the cancer cells. Psychological behaviors also play a major role in the mind's interaction with the body. This mind-body interaction strengthens the will to live. Training the mind can be a powerful advantage in maintaining health in the face of treatment side effects or in overall healing.

Dr. Susan Buchholz is available to the clinic's patients for an extensive regimen of psychological therapy focused on the healing process. She is certified in biofeedback which helps patients learn to control their body's activities more effectively through exercises monitored and reported by high technology instruments. She conducts personality analyses through the use of the Enneagram, a system that emphasizes spiritual development. Patients who may be depressed and distressed over their cancer prognosis learn to deal with their feelings and use that emotional energy in productive and healing ways. A healthy mind and spirit are keys to victory over cancer.

A local certified medical hypnotherapist is often called on to prepare Dr. Buchholz' patients for surgery, chemotherapy, and radiation through the use of guided imagery. He noted that the world's greatest athletes, particularly gymnasts, divers, and track stars, establish a mental image of exactly what they want to do. Through disciplined focus on that image, their body performs according to it. Cancer patients, through hypnosis, can do the same to discipline their body to do battle with their cancer cells and tolerate the conventional therapy.

Because we don't see a lot of headlines on clinical trials of integrative medicine, I looked forward to Dr. Buchholz' comments on statistical proof of its efficacy. He said that the difficulty of clinical trial confirmation of many complementary therapies is in the vast numbers of participants needed. Always hundreds, sometimes thousands, of patients must be willing to subject themselves to double-blind experiments for long periods of time. With relatively few integrative oncologists having relatively few patients to recommend for complementary therapy trials, such trials are limited. Add to that the general reluctance of the medical science community and government agencies to commit funds to tests outside the mainstream of medicine. The result is very little representation of complementary therapies in the clinical trial system.

He went on to say, however, that, notwithstanding the limited number of complementary medicine trials, integrative medicine has had some impressive successes. Surprisingly, the most convincing trial results have to do with physical exercise. Fitness activity has proven scientifically to help conventional therapies do their job and to ease side effects significantly. The next most scientifically proven natural therapy is spiritual practice. Prayer, meditation, and worship have been proven in many studies to reduce stress that inhibits healing and to strengthen the personal will that empowers the healing process. The third most scientifically confirmed complementary therapy is nutrition. Several clinical trials have concluded that certain foods, not isolated vitamins, have been shown to help prevent cancer. Selective whole foods have shown great promise as a cancer treatment complement, but there are still mixed results regarding food supplements. Clinical trials have been consistent in their findings that all commonly practiced complementary therapies increase the quality of life for patients going through cancer treatment.

When I asked why more oncologists are not becoming educated and experienced in integrative oncology, Dr. Buchholz enthusiastically countered that more are becoming interested. He went on to say it was regretful that there is still a public suspicion as well as a suspicion among medical professionals regarding integrative medicine. He believes more are practicing at least some types of complementary therapies than is being advertised. A lot of doctors, although convinced of its efficacy, are not ready to make it their brand label. For instance, they may give advice about certain natural complements to chemotherapy, but not publicly label themselves as an integrative oncologist.

Another factor that limits complementary therapy practice among oncologists is the sheer workload and expense that accompanies such a move. Most doctors are already suffering from work fatigue. Long hours with an excessive patient load do not create an environment that invites recommending, monitoring, and evaluating new and additional therapies. Integrative oncologists incur larger overheads to accommodate extra staff and equipment. Furthermore, the reluctance of health insurance companies to cover most complementary therapies places the integrative doctors in the position of being bill collectors. So, even with the generally lower costs of complementary therapies, the patient's inability to pay for the services and the insurance company's refusal to cover them create a financial dilemma for doctors. It is certainly easier and usually more profitable for a doctor to go with the flow of the mainstream disregarding complementary therapies.

I asked, then, what will convince the great majority of oncologists to pay the price, physically and financially, to become integrative in their practices?

Dr. Buchholz said plainly, "It's just a matter of economics. When patients start signing on with integrative doctors in greater numbers causing a loss of revenue for conventional-only doctors, those offering conventional-only will have to change."

My obvious next question was, "How do we bring about this change of behavior in cancer patients?"

"Like any other marketing effort," He answered. "We have to convince the public that integrative oncology has merit and should be considered in any comprehensive approach to cancer treatment. Your book will help significantly. Institutions like NIH, ACS, and medical schools will need to expand their focus to include more research of complementary therapies and integrative practice."

I requested Dr. Buchholz' long term vision for cancer treatment in America. I was expecting a long list of "to be accomplished" items. His was a simple three-point vision: a team process, an openness, and accountability.

A team process involving the oncologist, the patient, and complementary therapy practitioners will be necessary. The team would work in harmony with free flowing communication among all. The present prevailing model of the oncologist dictating, the patient blindly following, and any complementary therapy being done in isolation has to go. That model is insufficient at best and dangerous at worst.

Openness between the doctor and the patient will need to be paramount. The doctor must not withhold any knowledge of the patient's condition or options available. In turn, the patient must be totally transparent with the doctor and bold in expressing personal views and objectives. If anything is not understood by the patient, the patient should not let the doctor close the conversation. The patient should be candid about, and the doctor should be interested in, all aspects of the patient's life that bears on the healing process. This includes family situations, values, beliefs, financial priorities, fears, etc.

Accountability will need to be taken seriously on the part of both the doctor and the patient. The oncologist should accept ultimate responsibility for all therapies prescribed or recommended. He or she should lead the patient and manage the network of all therapies maintaining oversight of the entire process. The patient should be responsible for doing all he or she can do to maximize the treatment. For example, a cancer patient should not smoke or participate in any behavior that could jeopardize the treatment. All protocols agreed to should be followed by the patient with utmost discipline.

With a holistic approach to cancer treatment revolving around the principles of teamwork, openness, and accountability, the future of cancer treatment can be much brighter and promising.

As a final segment of the interview, I asked Dr. Buchholz to share any other personal thoughts about his practice that we had not touched on. He said he wanted to reiterate for my readers' understanding that he viewed integrative oncology from two different perspectives.

Some patients want every possible means of treatment to bring about every possible life-extending and healing opportunity. They readily accept appropriate conventional therapy—surgery, chemotherapy, and radiation. They collaborate with the oncologist and various complementary therapy providers for the greatest potential for maximum survival. For these patients, Dr. Buchholz helps define their goals for treatment, customizes the treatment to the individuals, and manages the treatments at the level agreed to by both him and the patients. The major objective of this approach is <u>longevity</u>.

Other patients want every possible means of treatment to bring about the least pain and most comfort as they deal with the disease. They may want some level of conventional therapy, but are mostly interested in what will keep their bodies most able to fight the disease naturally. They want to continue being whole and content. For these patients, Dr. Buchholz again helps define their goals and customizes treatment plans that both he and the patients agree to. The major objective of this approach is <u>quality of life</u>.

"I approach each patient in humility," Dr. Buchholz explained. "I listen intently to the patient's values and expectations, then combine that with my experience to recommend the best treatment plan that I can."

Knowing how rushed most doctors are with their overwhelming patient load, I asked how he could afford the time it must take to be so attuned to and focused on each patient. He said that some appointments only needed 15 minutes while others might require over an hour. His only criterion for appointment length is whatever it takes to know the patient. This concept of knowing the whole person as well as the sickness is a key principle of integrative medicine. It is one of the main differences that distinguish integrative from conventional practitioners.

Dr. William Buchholz, his wife, Dr. Susan Buchholz, and the staff of Buchholz Medical Group exemplify all that is right and good about integrative oncology. His practice is a template for the future of cancer treatment. The new strategy for the war on cancer will require this model of oncologist and oncology clinic to be accessible and affordable to all cancer patients.

CHAPTER 9

THE PATIENTS OF
INTEGRATIVE ONCOLOGY

Hopefully, you gained a lot of insight into the new strategy of integrative cancer treatment as you read through the last few chapters. Learning about new therapeutic methods, reviewing the historical progression of natural treatment pioneers, and reading about today's integrative medicine professionals have provided a broad panorama of where cancer treatment should be headed. Yet, there is no better perspective of integrative oncology than from the personal experience testimonies of those who have lived it. In this chapter, you will be invited into the lives of two cancer survivors who credit complementary therapies with saving their lives. Deciding on whom to interview among the myriads of cancer patients receiving complementary treatments was difficult. Rather than choosing those who might have best represented all integrative oncology patients, I settled on two who had significantly inspiring stories to tell. They had more onerous types of cancer than most others and less reason for hope.

Since the first person I interviewed was not the most likely candidate for integrative therapies, she contributes even more to the credibility of the strategy. She was a medical doctor with a very serious type of cancer who wasn't all that enthusiastic about complementary therapies. My other interview was with a gentleman who had "terminal" lung cancer and whose doctor told him he had only six months to live. Now, please enjoy and benefit from the stories of Maria Claudia and Frank.

Maria Claudia's Story

Maria Claudia White is a medical doctor in the specialty of immunology. She lives in Chapel Hill, North Carolina. As an immunologist, Dr. White is, of course, extremely conscious of her health. She has always been very disciplined in her diet of nutritious foods and in her use of supplemental vitamins and nutrients. Obviously, she has conscientiously kept her immune system at its peak. She had been the model doctor living an exemplary lifestyle of health and well being. Then, on September 19, 2008, her ob-gyn, Dr. Michele Quinn from Duke Medical Center, looked her in the eyes and said those life-altering words, "You have breast cancer."

Her instant reaction was all-consuming rage. This couldn't be happening to her. She was not just a physician—she was an *immunologist* for heaven's sake. Her whole profession was wrapped up in making sure people were taking care of their bodies and keeping them at superior ability to fight diseases. She didn't just talk the talk; she walked the walk. She ate organic foods, exercised, grew her own herbs and vegetables, didn't smoke or drink—not even coffee!

Dr. White soon learned that she carried the BRCAI gene mutation giving her a 60 to 80 percent greater likelihood of getting breast cancer and that, if contracted, it would be more aggressive. Worse yet, it was a triple-negative tumor which was not possible to be targeted with anti-estrogen, progesterone, or HER-2 therapies and was, therefore, more difficult to treat.

I learned of Dr. White's experience with complementary therapies from an article by Erin Quinn in *Natural Solutions* magazine and interviewed her after all treatments had been completed. I was not surprised to find that, although she was a prominent physician, she had limited knowledge of integrative oncology and complementary cancer treatments. She had no formal education or training in integrative medicine of any kind. I asked her what her level of awareness of complementary therapies was.

Claudia (her name preference) was aware that some oncologists recommended a healthy diet and use of vitamin supplements during chemotherapy and radiation therapies. She also knew about the recent tolerance advantages realized through biofeedback sessions during conventional treatment. However, the role other complementary therapies play in cancer recovery was a complete surprise. Her oncologist, Dr. Kimberley Blackwell, from Duke University Medical Center, recommended aggressive chemotherapy. But, along with this, she also recommended (more accurately, insisted on) a personalized regimen of complementary therapies available at Duke Integrative Medicine.

I asked how she chose her oncologist and whether she was aware of the oncologist's preference for integrative therapies.

Claudia said the surgeon who did her biopsy referred her to the oncologist. The recommended oncologist was renowned as a specialist in triple-negative breast cancers and for working closely with her patients. Claudia didn't know that she was also passionate about integrative oncology.

The first priority was to surgically remove a golf-ball size tumor near the lung. This was a complex and dangerous procedure that was conducted successfully. Next, a partial mastectomy on the left breast was performed followed by aggressive chemotherapy. Over the course of several months, Claudia suffered the typical hair loss from the chemotherapy. However, the complementary therapies, as I will reveal later, completely prevented or significantly reduced many of the side effects. Radiation was practically uneventful and, again, the accompanying natural therapies offset the negative reactions to a great extent. Claudia credits her success with the radiotherapy to a combination of skin care, exercise, nutrition, supplementation, and hypnotherapy.

I was curious about Claudia's first reaction to the recommended complementary therapies.

Without hesitation, she answered that she was very surprised and skeptical. Her physician at Duke Integrative Medicine, Dr. Evangeline Lausier, assessed Claudia's specific needs and urged her to accept five complementary therapies: nutrition and supplements, mind-body therapy, hypnotherapy, acupuncture, and biofeedback.

Claudia was fine with nutrition and supplements sessions, since she felt that she was already ahead of the curve in that area. And, knowing something about biofeedback, she was okay with that, too. Mind-body therapy was another story—a new frontier for her—and she considered it somewhat beyond the pale of rational thinking. Hypnotherapy? At first, she dismissed it completely. And, she was not eager in the least to try acupuncture, since she was afraid of needles (yes, a doctor afraid of needles).

Convincing Claudia to receive the complementary therapies was initially more of a challenge for her oncologist than was preparing her for the conventional therapies. Ultimately the oncologist prevailed by emphasizing the importance of these therapies in the healing process. The synergy between conventional and complementary therapies was presented to Claudia as the only hope for beating the formidable enemy of cancer. Because of the oncologist's relational approach to treating the whole person rather than just killing the tumor, she quickly gained Claudia's total confidence. The cancer treatment was a combined effort of both the doctor and patient. They were teammates in the healing challenge.

Nutrition and Supplements

I wanted to know how Claudia's eating habits changed after she began her sessions with her registered dietician, Beth Reardon, at Duke Integrative Medicine.

She indicated that what she ate didn't change dramatically, since she kept to a very healthy diet before her diagnosis. What changed was how she ate. Her dietician changed her eating schedule to small portions every two or three hours. This was to keep maximum nourishment in the blood stream 24/7 and to keep the glycemic levels constant since spikes in sugar levels during the day help feed the cancer. The normal American eating habit nourishes the cells for a few hours each day and starves them the rest of the time. A more frequent feeding protocol provides cancer-fighting sustenance to the body constantly.

The dietician periodically reviewed the records of Claudia's food intake to analyze what she seemed to be tolerating best during the treatment and made necessary adjustments to her plan. Some of the standard fare included herbal teas and an archetypical Mediterranean diet of fish, fruit, vegetables, whole grains, nuts, and olive oil.

Mind-body Therapy

"Exactly what did the mind-body therapy involve?" I asked.

"It was a comprehensive assessment of the interdependence of every aspect of my mind, body, and soul. My therapist caused me to look deeply inward, to realize my state of mind going into the conventional treatments. It was an effort to align my body and mind to facilitate such things as posture, respiration, meditation, relaxation, de-stress, and deep breathing."

She became keenly focused on these conditions rather than taking them for granted. It exercised her mind's ability to control her body by her command. This wasn't a lot of "touchy-feely" stuff, no chanting or new-age philosophies—just guided practice of mental concentration on the body.

Her anger about being a cancer victim was directed toward being angry with the cancer. She made images of the cancer tumor, then destroyed the images. She declared the tumor gone. She learned that worry was a form of meditation, but with concentration on the worst possible outcome. Her worry was changed to meditation on the best possible outcome. This relieved anxiety that interferes with the conventional therapy. Meditating on the positive actually increases the effectiveness of the conventional therapy.

Hypnotherapy

What Claudia was least confident in turned out to be one of her most beneficial therapies. She agreed to the hypnotherapy very reluctantly. It wasn't, as she had thought, having to subject herself to a trance of some kind. It was more of a suggestive thought exercise. Probably the primary benefit of hypnotherapy was pain reduction. Many of the side effects of surgery, chemotherapy, and radiation involve pain. A major portion of the hypnotherapy sessions was dedicated to obtaining a mental victory over pain—a denial of the pain. The hypnotherapy focused on amplifying the desired results and minimizing the negative ones. Claudia recalled that her thyroid surgery some years prior was followed by a very painful period of recovery. Her tumor surgery was more complex than the thyroid surgery, but she had hardly any pain associated with it.

She also told me about the typical reaction from radiotherapy that appears as a redness and burning sensation in the irradiated area. The hypnotherapist, Dr. Jeffrey Greeson, conducted some sessions with thought suggestions through which placing her hand in water and then on her breast would result in a lasting cooling sensation. He also coached her in visualizing a blue shield of temperature similar to the room temperature she had just placed in her hand. It worked, and she no longer experienced the burning. Each hypnotherapy session was recorded, and he asked her to download them to her iPod and listen to them on a daily basis just before falling asleep and, if possible, while sleeping.

Chemotherapy almost always causes a loss of taste and appetite. Claudia's hypnotherapy sessions dealt with that condition, and her appetite did not diminish. All food tasted like it should throughout her chemotherapy.

She also told me that, for quite some time after each session, her skin's redness would give way to her natural color, and the skin's elasticity would improve. She had no explanation for that other than it was her mind taking control of even the secondary side effects of the treatment.

Acupuncture

I joked with Claudia about her fear of needles and asked what convinced her to try acupuncture.

She said her oncologist told her that several studies show that acupuncture can minimize the side effects of chemotherapy, so she wanted her to have the acupuncture therapy. As a doctor, Claudia knew she needed to follow her doctor's advice. Ten sessions with the acupuncturist were set up prior to beginning her chemotherapy. The sessions were to prepare her body for the side effects of chemotherapy. She knew the principles of acupuncture, but didn't really understand why it worked.

In acupuncture, tiny needles are inserted into specific areas of the body to enhance blood flow and nerve response. This helps to relieve specific symptoms of the conventional treatment. Pain, stress, and anxiety are the targets of the acupuncture. Hot flashes and nausea from the chemotherapy are also reduced by the procedure.

Claudia said it made her feel better and gave her a clearer mind with which to cope with the treatments. Most people experience nausea for at least a week after each chemotherapy treatment. However, she said she was only slightly nauseated on the day of each treatment and had no lingering problem. She is convinced that her acupuncture treatments along with hypnotherapy helped her avoid the nausea and other side effects of chemotherapy. The acupuncturist noted that excessive mucous in her upper respiratory system could interfere with the chemotherapy, so he corrected that with strategically placed needles. Sure enough, the problem went away. Furthermore, a sense of well-being after each session resulted in a strong mindset of preparedness for the chemotherapy.

Biofeedback

Claudia's sessions with a biofeedback practitioner helped her to train her body to more efficiently process the conventional treatments and to evaluate how her body was responding to the treatments.

Biofeedback measures physiological activities through systematic monitoring of muscle tension, heart rate, skin conductivity, body temperature, breathing rate, etc. With the use of high-technology sensors, patients participate in certain exercises while viewing the results of their body's reactions in real time. Claudia learned to recognize what her body was doing in response to various conditions and to control its functions to a great degree. She learned how to modulate or reduce pain, anxiety, muscle tension, and gastrointestinal issues. The goal was to make her body work as efficiently as possible with as little interference in the treatment process and as much support of the healing process as possible. She began an aggressive physical exercise program requiring up to two hours each day of high-energy activity. The more she exercised, the better she felt. It was like a reprieve from the effects of the cancer and its treatment. Relaxation techniques were practiced seriously. There are special techniques to help the body to relax that she had never heard of. Both the exercise and relaxation had very positive effects on the brain and its ability to manage the body.

I was fascinated by Claudia's description of the biofeedback technologies.

Even from her perspective as a physician, she was impressed with the science involved in the processes. She explained that some of the machines worked like a highly sophisticated lie detector. She was asked questions and was given scenarios while connected to the monitors by various types of probes. The devices measured her temperature, blood pressure, hydration, and muscle tension. She viewed the monitors for real time feedback as to how her body was responding and was coached in how to control those responses.

I asked Claudia, "What was your greatest advantages from these sessions.

"I am certain that biofeedback was crucial to my stress management during treatment. I even changed the way I breathed. I determined what style of music soothed me most and prepared me best for my therapies and their side effects. My posture improved which allowed my body to perform with less restriction."

She said that, when fighting cancer, the body must have every advantage in the battle. Chemotherapy and radiation only work as well as they are accepted and supported by the body. She was more comfortable with the biofeedback sessions than any other complementary therapy and considers them the principal ingredient in her preparation and reception of the many challenges of cancer treatment.

The Overall Experience

Most patients subjected to conventional treatments find themselves overwhelmed by the burden of frequent treatment appointments. They often have to travel some distance to meet the challenging schedule while in a weakened and ill condition. I questioned Claudia about having to maintain both a conventional treatment schedule and the series of complementary therapies.

She described the complex schedule of therapies as very manageable. Every provider worked well with her to coordinate the sessions. The chemotherapy required the priority schedule, but she, her oncologist, and the Duke Integrative Medicine practitioners worked together as a team to set her appointments so as to allow the time necessary for the complementary treatments. It was like a seamless process blending as one series of treatments. She didn't think of it as a bunch of different commitments to keep track of, but rather as one set of treatments that integrated and flowed together nicely.

I asked Claudia to describe in just a few words the ultimate advantage of her complementary therapies.

She said that, if cancer therapy were described in terms of a war campaign, the conventional therapy would be the "shock and awe" part of the operation, and the complementary therapies would be the reconstruction—the offsetting of the conventional treatment. Most cancer patients describe the treatment as worse than the cancer. So, when the mind, body, and soul are consumed by the treatment, they cannot fight the cancer effectively. Complementary therapies such as those she received help to reserve the energies of the whole person to fight the cancer in conjunction with the conventional treatment. What sense is there in sending harsh chemicals and radiation into the body to attack the cancer, then letting your mind, body, and soul constantly battle those treatments? Complementary therapies prepare the mind, body, and soul to not only accept the treatments, but to collaborate with them to defeat the cancer. The combination forms a positive synergy that is absolutely essential for a full-scale assault on the disease.

I was interested in how her oncologist perceived the results of her complementary therapies.

"My oncologist could absolutely see the positive effects of the therapies. My physical stamina, attitude, pain tolerance, processing of the chemotherapy and radiation therapy, recovery from the surgery, and general sense of well being all contributed significantly to the success of the treatment. The complementary therapies also reduced the duration of the treatment."

I didn't want to get too personal, but needed to ask about her out-of-pocket costs for the complementary therapies.

Although she had adequate health insurance, few of the complementary therapies were covered by her policies. Through negotiations with her insurer, they paid for the acupuncture treatments and a few of the nutritional sessions.

Claudia lamented that, "Cost alone prohibits the advantages of integrative oncology for many cancer patients. I estimate paying over $3,000 per month for my complementary treatments. What a shame that something so essential to cancer treatment has to be such a financial burden or financially out of reach for most people."

My final question was how much of a role her complementary treatments played in her present state of remission.

"Absolutely key!" was her immediate response. Her type of cancer placed her in a statistically low chance of survival. It was highly aggressive and one of the most difficult categories to treat. Historically, the prognosis was not good for destroying BRACI triple-negative tumors. She is totally convinced that her cancer-free condition today is the result of the combined effort of the most modern conventional therapy complemented by the collective therapies specifically customized for her needs. Claudia was also quick to point out that the secondary benefits of the complementary therapies were that she avoided many of the debilitating and painful side effects normally suffered by conventional therapy patients, and that she learned skills and good habits that she can use for the rest of her life.

Of course, there are many other types of complementary therapies that are meticulously tailored to the varied needs of other cancer patients. Several of those have been described elsewhere in this book. Integrative oncologists are the experts in determining which therapies are most helpful for specific types of cancers and for particular people. What Claudia's oncologist prescribed was what Claudia needed.

Frank's Story

Franklin Whatley was a career school teacher. He took early retirement in his fifties to aid those of other cultures by teaching under-served students in rural communities. He and his wife, Nellie, moved from Oklahoma to Alaska for a few years where they experienced America's northern-most frontiers while pursuing their passion of teaching the disadvantaged. They later moved to Gallup, New Mexico, where they both taught in a school of predominantly Indian children.

It was 1993 during his first weeks in the New Mexico mountains that Frank noted some shortness of breath, but assumed it was because of the high altitude environment. He was sure his body would adjust to it. One day, tiring of a lingering cough and sore throat, Frank visited a Gallup doctor who prescribed cough syrup. After days of no relief from his symptoms, Frank returned to his doctor who ordered a chest X-ray. The film left no doubt as to the cause of the cough, sore throat, and shortness of breath. There, in the center of the picture, was a 10 centimeter spot on his left lung. The doctor immediately made him an appointment with a pulmonologist in Albuquerque.

Probably by divine appointment more than coincidence, Frank's and Nellie's son and his family were visiting them on the way to a new Army assignment. They provided comfort and perspective during this otherwise lonely time. The next day, both families dropped all plans and headed to Albuquerque.

The pulmonologist directed a CAT scan, but before the scan results were ready, Frank began spitting up blood. The scan showed the left lung blocked by the tumor which also appeared to be attached to the heart. The scan combined with the bleeding gave the doctor a clear diagnosis. His somber news: lung cancer, not operable, and a life expectancy of about six months.

After the doctor left the examining room, a dejected and defeated 58-year-old man turned to his wife and said, "Thirty-three years of marriage was not enough, was it?"

Late that the night on a motel bed, unable to sleep, Frank prayed, "God, if you take me in a few months, I will be the happiest fellow you ever saw when I get to Heaven. But, before I go, I will be the saddest fellow you ever saw. That's because I want to see my little grandson in the bed next to mine grow up along with all the grandchildren behind him." He paused, then he added, "But if that's not your will, it's okay with me."

The other children and grandchildren rushed to Albuquerque arriving just before Frank's bronchoscopy procedure which confirmed the diagnosis. In a quick family strategy meeting, everyone agreed that Frank and Nellie would return to Tulsa, the city they claimed as their home and where they still maintained a house. Within two days, they were on their way to Tulsa in an I-40 caravan of five cars and a rental truck loaded with their possessions. During their drive, a daughter-in-law announced that she was claiming the words of a bumper sticker she saw: *Expect a Miracle.*

"Let's just all expect a miracle for dad." she declared.

At Tulsa, a doctor friend recommended a cardiovascular surgeon and a pulmonologist. The surgeon believed that he could safely remove the lung and possibly extract the cancer. Frank encouraged his family with the hope that he could be cancer-free after the surgery. However, the surgery revealed the tumor was a squamous cell carcinoma with cells that had metastasized to the lymph nodes. The surgeon reported that, as he removed the lung, he had peeled part of the tumor off of the heart like peeling an orange. The doctors agreed that Frank should have aggressive chemotherapy and radiation.

The oncologist assigned to the case explained his plan to the family. There would be radiation followed by aggressive chemotherapy. The Whatley's daughter, LaNell, was a registered nurse and had many questions. Would the radiation procedures ensure that the body would have maximum protection from the effects of the harmful rays? Would there be a port inserted into the body for the chemotherapy—a relatively new technique at the time? What diet would be recommended, and what supplements would be prescribed? The answers were disappointing. Little radiation protection was available, this hospital didn't use ports for chemotherapy, cancer patients could eat about anything they wanted, and supplements were not needed.

At that point, LaNell insisted that her dad go to a Cancer Treatment Centers of America (CTCA) hospital nearby where integrative oncologists practice complementary therapies including special nutrition and supplement protocols. CTCA also used the latest state-of-the-art protection for radiation therapy and the new chemotherapy ports. Their treatment philosophy was to do as little harm as possible to the body, to build up the body's natural immune system, and to depend on a holistic approach to healing the whole person. Treating the disease included treating the body and spirit as well.

Upon hearing about the plan to use CTCA in Tulsa, the daughter-in-law who claimed the bumper sticker statement began to realize its significance even more. The facilities that housed Tulsa's CTCA Southwest Regional Medical Center at that time were owned by the Oral Roberts organization whose motto was *Expect a Miracle.*

"That's it," she exclaimed to the family. "Expect a miracle in the Oral Roberts building!"

I was caught up in this fascinating story as I sat with Frank and Nellie at the dining table in the relaxed atmosphere of their home seventeen years later. The three of us crunched on nachos and cheese followed by Nellie's delicious homemade snicker doodle cookies. The tape recorder was consuming every word, and I was feverishly scribbling commentary notes. I paused to ask what they noticed as the difference in conventional and integrative treatment when they switched to the integrative treatment center.

Frank smiled and said, "I could feel it when I walked into the hospital. They were friendly. They treated me with respect. They were always wanting to help with directions, answering questions, and providing whatever I needed. Everyone seemed so positive. I didn't feel rushed in anything I was doing unlike the case in most other medical facilities. Once I met people, they always remembered my name."

At an orientation meeting, department heads clearly presented what could be expected in the treatment process. Question and answer periods were very helpful. Toward the end of the meeting, an executive explained that those present who survived five years would be presented a live tree to plant on the hospital campus in a special tree planting ceremony. The tree would be a living tribute to their success in gaining victory over cancer. After that announcement, Frank voiced loudly, "Get my tree ready!"

I inquired about his first meeting with his new integrative oncologist. He said he actually had two oncologists, one radiation oncologist, Dr. James Flynn, and one chemotherapy oncologist, Dr. Hans Nivenny. They coordinated the plans for his treatment and made sure he understood and agreed with every aspect of it. The radiation would be highly concentrated on a very small area. The rest of the body would be covered with a lead shielding apparatus that would make sure that no other area would be touched by the radiation. The chemotherapy would be infused by "infractionated" doses. These low-intensity, higher frequency doses of chemotherapy avoided the shock of the larger amounts of toxic chemicals on the body. They also balanced the levels of the chemicals in the body over a longer period without a break in effectiveness. Instead of the typical heavy, hour-long chemotherapy infusions one to three times a week, Frank was given much smaller, more manageable infusions over a period of 12 hours each day for five consecutive days. With three-week breaks between the one-week infusions, his chemotherapy took eight months. His radiation therapy was administered over a six-week period.

The radiation and chemotherapy were accompanied by very few side effects. There was almost no nausea except for the first round of chemotherapy, and he maintained a healthy appetite. Amazingly, instead of losing weight, he gained 35 pounds during treatment. Although he did lose his hair temporarily, the lower dose, longer duration therapy seemed to preclude many of the painful, aggravating, and physically distressing problem that plague most of those receiving exclusively conventional therapies.

Nutrition and Supplements

A vital part of the treatment regimen was regular sessions with the center's nutritionist, Patrick Quillin, PhD. Recall Dr. Quillin from Chapter 5, a prolific writer and scientist in the field of cancer and nutrition. At these sessions, Dr. Quillin and his staff instructed the Whatleys in the best choices of menus during various phases of their treatment. His office monitored their progress and motivated them to eat right. Many cancer-treatment-unique recipes and techniques were offered for preparing fresh fruits, vegetables, whole grain products, etc. for mealtime.

The nutrition department also prescribed specific nutritional supplements to be taken on a rigid schedule that complemented the patient's therapy schedule. Frank's individualized prescription involved 13 different supplements.   He continues to this day to take supplements from the nutrition department of CTCA with all discipline.

Most of CTCA's patients were in-patients for much of their treatment, since the treatments often lasted all day, every day. Therefore, much of their diet was from hospital food which was very tasty and unquestionably nutritious. At any time during the day or night, snacks were available in the cafeteria. This perk included organic fruits, vegetables, and other healthy foods. Immune system boosting herbal teas and juices were also available at convenient locations throughout the hospital.

Spiritual Support

As is the case for most integrative oncology centers, CTCA considers the spiritual welfare of the whole person to be crucial to success in the healing process. A chaplain was on the premises 24/7 and routinely visited and prayed with the patients. Scheduled worship, prayer, and devotional times were part of the weekly schedule. A variety of support groups were available for sharing and encouragement. The staff fostered close relationships among the patients. In just a few days, patients would know each others' names and backgrounds. One-on-one spiritual counseling could be requested. Family counseling was promoted with the understanding that close family relationships were essential to physical healing. A principle of integrative oncology is that, although the medical practitioners will do all they can to care for the patient, it is ultimately the family who will provide most of the care. It is important to make sure they are trained and equipped properly. Anyone who desired to attend services at a local church in the community was provided transportation to do so. When patients left the center, they were urged to continue to give priority attention to the spiritual realms of their lives. Both Frank and Nellie received much comfort and hope from this element of the treatment.

Physical and Recreational Therapy

Frank often took advantage of the full-service gym. Exercise equipment and an indoor walking track provided ample opportunity for maintaining as much physical fitness as possible with the therapies. Integrative oncologists will almost always insist that their patients do as much physical exercise as they can to keep muscles toned and the cardiovascular system at peak.

Even competitive sport options were offered. For example, pool tables were for patient recreation, family activity, and "serious" tournaments. Frank said that the staff was adamant that patients stay active during their therapy and never become couch potatoes even when they felt physically drained.

Patients or their family members who were somewhat crafty had outlets for displaying, trading, or selling their crafts. Certain areas were reserved for mini-craft fairs and filled with projects that patients or their loved ones worked on during treatment. Promoting the productivity of any patient has always been a principal objective of integrative medicine.

Nellie mentioned the special events that everyone looked forward to. There were theme nights and sing-alongs. Dr. Quillin, the nutritionist, sometimes played his guitar and sang country music. It was always fun to see the highly professional doctors with a passion for treating cancer ham it up with the patients and families during these times.

The Insurance Issue

The decision about choosing integrative cancer treatment, or any kind of integrative care for that matter, always gets to the financial question. I asked Frank about that.

"It was more expensive," he admitted. "But, we were committed to do whatever it took. It was that important."

He confided that he had a rather good insurance plan. The most expensive therapies, of course, were radiation and chemotherapy. Then there were the hospital and individual doctor costs. All of those services were billed to the insurance company, and the Whatleys paid the deductibles and out-of-pocket costs. The services of the nutritionist, the special diets during outpatient care, and the supplements were not covered by insurance. Likewise, post treatment supplements have not been covered. Sadly, the insurance shortfall keeps many patients from having the advantage of quality integrative cancer treatment.

The Rest of the Story

To borrow the late Paul Harvey's line, the proof of success in Frank's integrative oncology experience is in "the rest of the story."

On May 7, 1999, five years after his treatment, Franklin Whatley, took a shovel, made a hole in the ground, and planted a tree on the campus of the cancer center that he says saved his life. He stood with several other five-year cancer survivors who, on that day, celebrated their new lease on life. In doing so, they also celebrated a budding future for a new brand of cancer treatment, a new strategy that has been long overdue and not yet recognized widely enough. Today, on the grounds of Cancer Treatment Centers of America's Southwestern Regional Medical Center, there stands a tree in honor of a man who believed God was going to give him a long and fruitful life in spite of the six-month death sentence. He also believed the best chance for that to happen was with treatment that offered more than the traditional approach.

I asked Frank what he thought his future would have been like if he had stayed with his original exclusively conventional treatment program in 1993.

"I wouldn't have been here today." he answered, simply.

Then he continued, "Let me give you just one example of why I think that's true. A neighbor of mine had almost the same diagnosis of lung cancer that I had. He chose the conventional route with no complementary therapies. We had the same type of radiation therapy. He later had a heart attack that required heart bypass surgery. When the doctors got to his heart, it was burned by the past radiation beyond being repaired. They sewed him back up without accomplishing anything, and he died three months later."

Frank explained further, "Then, I had a heart attack in my sixties that required surgery. My heart surgeon initially refused to do the surgery because I had received radiation therapy for cancer. My radiation technologist at CTCA convinced my heart surgeon that my heart had been protected from my radiation therapy. The heart surgeon finally agreed to do the surgery and told me afterward that my heart was not damaged in any way by the radiation."Frank went on to say that, not only did the integrative oncology treatment heal him from cancer, but the precautions taken during the treatment allowed him to survive two heart attacks.

After treatment, Frank had thorough follow-up checkups every three months. Checkups became longer spaced from year to year. Now, he has one checkup a year. Since the last day of treatment, nothing suspicious has ever appeared. At the time of my interview, he was 74 years old.

Sadly, though, the family did have cancer strike again. Their daughter, LaNell, was recently diagnosed with breast cancer. She is scheduled for a radical mastectomy at CTCA. She has the same positive attitude and hope that her father demonstrated. In preparation for her surgery, the hospital required her to refrain from sodas, chocolate, caffeine, and nicotine for two weeks. She doesn't smoke, but the other three restrictions were accepted commitments although not welcomed. She has also been placed on a strict nutritional supplement regimen.

Such preparation is hardly ever required by hospitals that do not offer integrative medicine care.

The commitment of this family to integrative cancer treatment is phenomenal. LaNell is classified as a Cherokee Indian which allows her co-pay to be covered for treatment in a Bureau of Indian Affairs network hospital. This would mean all medical care would be provided without patient cost for those insured. Integrative oncology hospitals and practitioners are not in that network. LaNell, with the support of her family, will choose to forego conventional cancer treatment at no cost to her in favor of paying for integrative treatment. They have experienced the future of cancer treatment and refuse to turn back regardless of the costs and circumstances.

LaNell will fortunately have further advantages that her father didn't have seventeen years ago. CTCA now provides numerous other complementary treatments that have proven successful in recent years such as acupuncture, naturopathic medicine, mind-body medicine, image enhancement, and chiropractic care.

Remember Frank's first words after hearing his death sentence: "Thirty-three years of marriage wasn't enough, was it?" Well, before the year of this interview ends, the Whatleys will celebrate their Golden Wedding Anniversary! They have already made plans to have a party in the CTCA hospital. Frank said that would be only appropriate because, "If we hadn't gone to CTCA, we wouldn't have had a 50th."

As we closed the interview, Nellie brought out a scrapbook of their time at CTCA. It would have won first place at a scrapbooking club contest. It looked more like a pictorial archive of a family vacation than a record of cancer treatment. I thought as I perused the photos how I wished every victim of cancer could have this kind of experience and outcome. One day soon.

I gathered my material together after having spent the most uplifting few hours in recent memory with these folks. What a gracious, hospitable, and brave family. We hugged, said our good-byes, and promised to keep in touch.

As I started to leave, Frank said, "Oh, here, you might want to take a snack for your flight back." He handed me a plastic bag filled with those awesome snicker doodle cookies.

A Final Thought

Claudia's and Frank's experiences should be that of every cancer patient. Sadly, their experience is extremely rare. Of over 12 million patients undergoing cancer treatment or monitoring in the United States at any given time, probably no more than a few thousand are realizing the benefits of any kind of complementary therapy under the care of a professional practitioner. The vast majority of cancer sufferers have no idea what integrative oncology even is. Most of those that are knowledgeable of it find it unfeasible due to travel distance or cost. This is a travesty for citizens of the richest nation in the world with the best medical system in the world. We must settle for no less than a complete strategy overhaul for cancer treatment. However, the opposition and challenges to such a strategy overhaul are real and formidable as you will see in the next four chapters.

PART 3

THE NEW STRATEGY CHALLENGES

CHAPTER 10

THE POLITICAL FACTOR

When most people would judge the exclusive practice of conventional medicine as failing to make reasonable progress in the war against cancer, we have to ask what is wrong. When we consider what little has been done and is being done in expanding our horizons beyond sole reliance on conventional medicine, we have to ask why. When we see so much money being spent on conventional efforts that have a questionable track record while so few resources go toward promising integrative options, we have to wonder how that is happening. When we consider the passions and skills of integrative oncologists and the positive experiences of their patients, we are perplexed that everyone isn't moving in that direction.

America has the most advanced medical technology in the world. It has the most thoroughly educated, most highly trained, and most dedicated medical professionals in the world. It infuses more money into medical research and infrastructure than any other country in the world. We have to conclude that the lack of progress in cancer treatment is not a capability issue, not a motivational issue, not a science issue, and not a resources issue. Then what is it?

In a word: it is <u>politics</u>.

My dictionary defines politics as *"competition between competing interest groups or individuals for power and leadership in government or other group."* As unproductive and divisive as it is, conflict seems to always exist among people who have a critical interest in major life-impacting goals. Perhaps after religion and government, medical care has a greater impact on the lives of people than any other institution. The who, what, when, and where questions accompanying the need for medical care are usually emotionally charged and subject to strong opinion. We recently saw the government's attempt to reform health care polarize the entire nation. People on both sides of the issue were screaming at each other in town hall meetings.

Money is almost always a significant factor in the debate. Medical care is costly and commands the attention of both the payer and the payee. In 2008, Americans spent 17% of the Gross Domestic Product (GDP) on medical care—almost twice the average of the 10 leading industrialized nations. That equated to $2.4 trillion total or $7,900 for every man, woman, and child (Centers for Medicare and Medicaid Services 2008). That money comes out of the pockets of families and insurance companies and is poured into the pockets of medical and pharmaceutical practitioners and institutions. It generates huge competitive pressures among the players in that market.

Competition appropriately applied in business is good and is the foundation of our free market capitalist economy. Usually, competition ensures that the best products and services prevail. It is only when the government or other controlling powers interfere with the free flow of products and services that the market becomes skewed. When consumers lose the right to decide on what they can or cannot purchase, a free market economy ceases to exist. When producers and entrepreneurs lose the right to make available to consumers what will satisfy the consumers, a free market economy ceases to exist. If either of these conditions is present in a certain sector of the market, such as medical care, a free market in that sector ceases to exist. In the United States, a free market does not exist in medical care.

Of course, we must have a certain amount of regulatory systems that prevent fraudulent products and services from harming unsuspecting consumers. Drug producers must be made to prove that they are not offering the afflicted something that could be either useless or more harmful than good. Medical practitioners must be required to have proper education and licenses. Health facilities, both educational and clinical, must be accredited and regularly inspected. No one would argue the need to maintain these types of safeguards. Sadly, political influence in American medicine projects itself well beyond these standards. There is a political bias favoring exclusive conventional medicine and opposing non-pharmacological medicine that probes much more deeply into the free market than necessary. For decades, this bias has supported the biggest institutions of the medical and pharmaceutical industries while stifling most of the efforts of non-pharmacological medicine researchers and entrepreneurs.

Our Prescription Culture

Although non-pharmacological medicine is making some progress slowly into the mainstream, we are still very much a divided society of "official" versus "unofficial" medicine. Toxic and debilitating cancer treatments are pushed to the forefront of modern medicine by the medical establishment. Potentially effective non-toxic options, even as integrative and complementary protocols, are usually rejected without the benefit of free market competition. The medical establishment or institutions which control the politics of this virtually closed market include the U.S. Food and Drug Administration (FDA) and the American Medical Association (AMA). The National Institutes of Health (NIH) with its National Cancer Institute (NCI) also plays a major role in public opinion of what is acceptable in cancer treatment. Other very influential institutions include the American Cancer Society (ACS) and mega cancer centers such as M.D. Anderson, Memorial Sloan Kettering, and the Mayo Clinic. The FDA and AMA, through regulations and policy, virtually control which medicines and treatments are available and which are prohibited. They have enforcement authority and control the licensing of medical professionals and facilities. The entire medical field in America is subject to their rules and disciplinary actions. They dictate that doctors can only prescribe certain medicines—often harsh chemicals with side effects—and certain procedures. They also have a lot to do with what insurance companies will cover, effectively limiting what is affordable to consumers.

Here is the irony. According to the *Journal of the American Medical Association* (JAMA), the fourth leading cause of death in American hospitals is from reactions to the "official" drugs approved, promoted, and issued by the medical establishment (JAMA 1998). The JAMA published in 1998 a shocking report after a 30-year study. The report showed that 106,000 people a year die in hospitals from FDA-approved drugs. That is one death every five minutes. The number of deaths from prescription drugs is exceeded only by that of heart disease, cancer, and stroke. When including those dying outside of hospitals, such as in the home, the number of deaths annually rises to 140,000, or about one every four minutes. This is three times the number of deaths from automobile accidents. Furthermore, the fourth leading cause of hospital admissions in America is from reactions to FDA-approved prescription drugs (USA Today 1998). Recent studies show that we Americans spend slightly more on treating the adverse effects of prescription drugs than we spend on the drugs themselves (Light Party 2008). These statistics have nothing to do with illegal street drugs which cause far fewer deaths and hospital admissions than legal drugs.

This risk from approved drugs is also clearly evident from the lucrative market that drug-related incidents have created for the lawyers. Numerous law firms specialize in monitoring legal drugs for potential serious side effects or deaths from their use. They have found plenty of opportunities to rally those who have been harmed by the drugs and represent them in individual or class action lawsuits. The race between car dealers pushing cars and law firms seeking drug victims seems to be tightening for dominance of TV commercial time.

The United Nations World Health Organization (WHO) reports statistics on its member countries, one of which is termed "healthy life expectancy." This category is defined as the number of years a person is expected to live in a healthy condition with times of illness subtracted from the life span. The latest WHO report ranks the U.S. at number 25 behind all of Europe and other major countries like Canada, Japan, and Australia (WHO 2008). In other words, the people of 24 other industrialized nations live more healthy years than Americans. Yet, the report lists our country as the highest spender on conventional health care of any member country as a percentage of gross domestic product. So, U.S. citizens spend more on their medical care than citizens of almost all major industrialized countries, but get fewer healthy years of life for their money.

The United Kingdom does an annual report on international health comparisons. This report includes statistics on the deaths per 100,000 people from all cancers in the ten leading industrialized nations. These cancer mortality rates range from 152 to 189 (National Audit Office 2008). The United States is unimpressively in the upper part of the range at 181. Again, we Americans spend much more than citizens of any other major country on cancer prevention and treatment while experiencing a higher than average death rate from the disease.

The culture of health care that we Americans have evolved into is a religious-like confidence in highly complex, expensive chemically engineered pharmaceuticals and super technical medical procedures. Considering the money that we dole out to cure everything from sore throats to cancer, we should expect the best results in the world. We have heard medical pundits argue often that the expense is worth it to have access to the best health care on the globe. This argument usually accompanies a debate on out-of-control health care costs. Well, according to numerous statistics, we do not have the best health care on the globe from a cost-benefit perspective.

Now, I will offer a qualification that we do have fine facilities and equipment in this country. Almost everything about institutionalized medicine in America looks good on the surface compared to most other countries. Our hospitals are immaculate and inviting. That is a very positive aspect of our medical culture. And, there is no doubt in my mind that we have experienced many pharmaceutical and methodological breakthroughs that have saved innumerable lives and vastly improved qualities of lives. The question is why are we so myopic in our view of medicine that we will not broaden our acceptance of opportunities outside the mainstream, particularly those that would reduce costs? Why are we not researching an abundance of simpler, natural, less costly options that show great potential? Other industrialized countries have embraced a myriad of natural medicines and less-intrusive practices and are reporting better results than we are because of it.

Our dependence on prescription drugs and conventional medicine has made health care the largest industry in the country. In order to benefit from it, we are controlled by it. What the industry makes available is our only option. We pay the price set by the industry because the industry is virtually monopolistic. Although there is some competition within the industry, it is not a free market. In the food industry, if you don't like the prices, you can eat less or plant a garden. In the transportation industry, if you can't afford a new vehicle, you can choose a used one, ride a bike, or stay home. You are free to choose based on your resources, priorities, and preferences. Conversely, in the health care industry, you have hardly any choices. Generally, if you have cancer in this country, you can't ask your doctor for a more affordable type of treatment. You usually can't ask him or her for a less harmful treatment. You can't even ask for his or her assistance in your self treatment. If you want to choose a remedy that shows great promise, but that is not "official" medicine, your doctor will seldom accommodate you. Your doctor will not let you choose, because he or she could lose his or her license and likely commit a crime in doing so. Your doctor, with few exceptions, can only prescribe traditional, conventional treatments at exorbitant prices with lower than acceptable success rates. Many oncologists will not even consider recently approved integrative treatment because it is not considered mainstream. How did we in America, the greatest society in human history, fall into this conundrum?

A History of Frustration

It is quite a paradox that a nation founded on the values of life, liberty, and the pursuit of happiness finds little of the three reflected in its approach to health care. Regarding life, the U.S. accepts a cancer mortality rate no lower than most other highly developed countries. Regarding liberty, it controls its doctors' practices and prescriptions, by regulation, policy, or culture more restrictively than most other places in the world. Regarding the pursuit of happiness, its citizens have less control over their treatment choices than almost anyone anywhere else. Our state of health care, especially cancer treatment, did not become this way overnight. It has evolved over a century and a half of big business profiteering, bureaucratic stifling, and political power plays.

Cancer treatment has become a culture of its own. What we are dealing with now is not based on the deliberate thoughts and actions of professionals in the cancer industry as they pursue their daily responsibilities. We know that every individual in the cancer fighting profession wants nothing more than to see the disease defeated. They are all simply products of an environment that has standards and strategies established by the most powerful secular influences on earth. The institutions of medicine, pharmaceutics, and government form a train that is seemingly unstoppable. Now that this express train that moves the largest industry in America has reached cruise speed, everyone on it—practitioners and patients alike—are just along for the ride.

Let me make doubly sure I am being clear here. I don't believe that anyone in the cancer treatment industry has the personal objective of subverting a cure for cancer or of deliberately harming a patient unnecessarily. A researcher in a prominent cancer center doesn't prejudice a lab experiment in order to disqualify a potentially effective natural medicine. An oncologist doesn't withhold information on non-toxic treatment from a patient because she wants to make more money. A pharmaceutical executive doesn't sit at his desk thinking of new ways to keep bona fide competitive products off the market. A medical school professor doesn't stand before his class and knowingly teach ineffective medicine. An elected government official doesn't knowingly cast a vote that will prevent a cancer cure. I can't point a finger at any individual, or any group of individuals and say there is why we are not making headway against cancer. The problem is much larger than that. It is an institutional culture that been building for many decades. Before we can expect to succeed in any change of the cultural course at all, we have to know something of its history and why it is what it is.

When sincere missionaries begin a new work in an unfamiliar part of the world, they begin by learning the people, their culture, and their history. Until those with the truth know what made unbelievers who they are, they can't expect to show them a new direction. Likewise, proponents of a new cancer strategy can't expect to change the minds of advocates of conventional-only treatment without understanding where they are coming from. So, let's embark on a brief historical journey of the who's and what's of cancer treatment.

The I.G. Farben Company

In 1926, a German industrialist named Hermann Schmitz and a Swiss banker named Eduard Greutert partnered to form a company they called I.G. Farben. I.G. Farben, roughly translated from German Deutsch means "chemical cartel." The vision of Schmitz and Greutert was to grow a company that would ultimately dominate the world chemical market, and they had the resources and influence to do it. By the beginning of World War II, the company had already become the largest industrial enterprise in Europe and the largest chemical company in the world. Within just a few years, I.G. Farben owned or controlled most chemical companies in Europe. It also formed strategic partnerships with numerous United States corporations such as Alcoa, Atlantic Oil, Bell and Howell, Dow Chemical, DuPont, Eastman Kodak, Goodyear, Gulf Oil, Monsanto Chemical, Proctor and Gamble, Standard Oil, and Texaco. It purchased outright or a controlling interest in Bayer Company, Sterling Drug Company, Van Ess Laboratories, Merrill Company, Bristol Meyers, Squibb Pharmaceutical, and scores of other American chemical, drug, and petroleum companies (Griffin 1997).

As monopolies and cartels in other parts of the world were learning, I.G. Farben's survival would depend on its power and influence over the government of its homeland. They could only continue market domination as long as they could infiltrate the top levels of government and move it in a more centralized direction. Monopolies can only thrive in a dictatorial or socialist government where they can be protected from free trade and the will of the consumer. As Adolph Hitler rose to power, much of his support came from I.G. Farben and other German cartels. Fascist Germany was in large measure thriving by monopolists control over the government. The government, in turn, favored the monopolists and prevented competition.

In the months leading up to the U.S. entry into World War II, many of the top American corporations found themselves in a major dilemma. Their connections with I.G. Farben were dependent on the free flow of trade with the now Nazi Germany industrial giant. Many of the patents for their products were held by the company that was now supplying Germany's military. I.G. Farben was demanding the continuance of exports from the U.S. to Germany, but was not reciprocating. The success of the U.S. companies depended on international trade with their German parent company or major partner. I.G. Farben was largely flourishing from the technology and productivity of U.S. companies. Secret international meetings were being conducted. Much of corporate America and corporate Germany was in a tightly wound state of stress.

As the U.S. entered the war, the monolithic corporations on both sides of the Atlantic agreed to refocus on their respective governments' call to arms and to a temporary hiatus in their partnerships. The assumptions were that relationships would be back to normal after the war driven by fiscal reality. Everything considered, this was all a big win-win for corporate America and I.G. Farben. International exports and imports up to the eve of the war helped both nations spin up each other's industrial base and war making capability. During the war, each company profited greatly from its own government. Probably not one executive in any of the companies ever thought that he or she was leading the company to aid the enemy by financially benefiting from exports of war-making products and technology. Yet, industries just continued to trade internationally with unrestrained momentum, each side helping the other prepare for war of unprecedented scale.

Please indulge me in a short excursion here to consider a point of analogy. Some may think it a quantum leap to view the impact of big business on World War II as reflecting conventional medicine's impact on the war against cancer. But, I believe there is similarity and a lesson to be learned here. The powerhouses of corporate America continued business as usual with the enemy when they should have been changing strategies to thwart its expansion. I often hear comments like, "The greatest medical system in the world can't be on the wrong track when it comes to dealing with cancer." Or, "The best minds and the finest institutions in the history of medicine just need more time and more of our support to find the cure." Could what is happening in the war against cancer be analogous to what happened in World War II? Could health care conglomerates and pharmaceutical giants be so preoccupied with what has been profitable that they conveniently overlook what is happening outside their sphere of operation? Could our unrestrained dependence on the momentum of big medicine be actually harming the fight by giving advantage to the enemy—cancer? Back to the story.

Within just a few months after the war, corporate America was scrambling to reconnect with German industry according to prewar terms. In many cases, company names and executive faces had changed, but the money and the market was inviting attention. U.S. firms were hungry to get back to what was working so well before. They were largely the energy behind reconstruction of the German economy. The early post-war years ushered in the rise of the dominant corporations that would become the drivers of the world economy for the foreseeable future. For decades to come, the U.S. would be the hub of business and economic activity as its major corporations led the world market. Corporations were forming cartel-like combinations that mirrored the pre-war models. This was the era that launched the U.S. into position as the most powerful nation in human history. Every American citizen born since the forties has benefited immensely from this explosion of corporate and political influence. However, it brought with it a certain loss of individual and entrepreneurial freedom. For over a half century, big business has tended to stifle or ignore the creative and innovative contributions of individuals and smaller organizations outside of their realm. New ideas and products are too often invalidated as incompatible with the objectives of the mainstream industrial complex. If recommendations are not generated from within the official bureaucratic networks, they are easily discarded. Nowhere has this atmosphere been more prevalent than in the health care industry.

Big Business, Big Pharma, and the FDA

If you were asked what name comes to mind first when you think of big business history in America, you would likely say, Rockefeller. It makes no difference what era of our industrial history you consider, early 19th century to present. It makes no difference which Rockefeller you reference, William, John D., John D., Jr., or David and his siblings. For over a century, the name Rockefeller has dominated the burgeoning realm of industry in America. The automobile had hardly made its debut before Rockefeller family established Standard Oil Company of New Jersey. Standard Oil became the holding company for many other domestic and foreign oil companies. Likewise, the family, by the mid-1900's, formed The Chase Manhattan, the largest banking firm in the world. The deposits of Chase Manhattan have consistently amounted to more than the annual budgets of most nations. It would be difficult to find many large businesses in this country or abroad that are not associated in some way with a Rockefeller enterprise.

Before continuing, I want to declare that I am not anti-business. I am not even anti-big-business. My degrees are in business, and I teach business courses at the university level. I acknowledge and appreciate the extraordinary contributions that our country's leading corporations have made in establishing the affluence and amenities that we as a society enjoy. Neither am I anti-government. Our government has led us to the position of the most formidable and envious nation on earth. It secures that position for us with unprecedented democracy and freedom. The bureaucracy of both big business and big government is generally unavoidable and a necessary inconvenience in exchange for its benefits. I was part of that institutional bureaucracy for most of my adult life in the upper levels of the military. I understand it well. The super rich icons of big business and the powerful politicians of big government are in large measure responsible for and deserve credit for the remarkable society in which we have the joy of living. The interactions and interdependence of American business and government have been the catalyst for the life, liberty, and pursuit of happiness that we cherish. Regardless of one's opinion of the recent bailouts and bridge loans the government gave to big business, it demonstrated just how critical collaboration of both institutions is to our economic survival. So, as I appraise the role of big business and big government in the way our society deals with cancer treatment, it is not from a disdain or ignorance of the establishment. It is from my passion to urge the establishment to change its approach to this particular problem.

The movement of key leaders in the nation's top banking and pharmaceutical industry into the offices of major government agencies is intriguing. Former Secretaries of State John Foster Dulles and Dean Rusk were heads of the Rockefeller Foundation. Former Secretary of the Treasury, Douglas Dillon was on the board of the Chase Manhattan Bank. John J. McCloy, President of the UN World Bank was previously Chairman of the Board of the Chase Manhattan and trustee of the Rockefeller Foundation as well as Chairman of the Executive Committee for Squibb Pharmaceutical. President Richard Nixon and Attorney General John Mitchell were Wall Street attorneys for Warner-Lambert Pharmaceutical.

The fraternal network of some of the most influential people in the world has created the relatively closed circles of big finance, big chemical/pharmaceutical, and big government. "Big pharma" is a commonly used term to describe the few mega-corporations that produce most modern drugs and medical equipment. It doesn't take much research to confirm that big pharma has been inextricably linked to the world's largest financial institutions and highest political offices. These interrelationships produce strong mutual support for the interests of each realm. Politicians depend on contributions and influence from big business, especially pharmaceuticals. Big finance and big pharma depend on favorable government legislation. As long as stock holders of big finance and big pharma demand maximum profits, and as long as politicians need contributions and taxes, these three will continue to be bed partners, sometimes at the expense of the public.

Although the Rockefeller family and many other business empires were built within the environs of America's free market capitalism, their immeasurable acquisitions and powerful political influence significantly affected the entire international economy. David Rockefeller, speaking at a world investment forum, told international investment leaders that it was wise to invest in "life and risk insurance companies, business equipment companies, and companies benefiting from research into drugs." (Griffin 1997) Subsequently, he and his family have followed that advice. Their influence and the influence of their colleagues continue to dominate the chemical and pharmaceutical markets. Almost all drug producers in the U.S. today got their start through the fortunes of the Rockefellers, the Carnegies, the Mellons, or the Morgans. Big business influence in pharmaceuticals has kept it one of the least competitive markets in the free world. If not monopolies, the huge corporations that make almost all of our drugs certainly comprise cartel-like market segments that coordinate production and strategies. The result is virtual control over the drug industry by a relatively few companies, many of which are subsidiaries of even fewer parent companies.

Of the top 10 pharmaceutical companies in the world in 2009, five were in the U.S. as depicted in Table 10-1 (Contract Pharma 2009). Almost half of the world's market share and total sales of drugs are from the U.S. big pharma companies. The American pharmaceutical industry, consisting of just a handful of tremendously powerful corporations, has substantial influence in the strategy and direction of the world's prescription drug market including cancer treatment drugs. The industry has overwhelming momentum and little incentive to be swayed.

Table 10-1   Top 10 Pharmaceutical Companies in Sales

Companies	Sales (Millions)
1. Pfizer*	$44,174
2. Sanofi-Aventis	$40,562
3. GlaxoSmithKline	$37,810
4. Novartis	$35,647
5. AstraZeneca	$30,677
6. Merck*	$25,901
7. Johnson & Johnson*	$24,567
8. Roche	$23,624
9. Eli Lilly & Co.*	$19,285
10. Bristol-Myers Squibb*	$17,715

* American companies

Now, let's do a little deductive thinking. The U.S. is home to half of the top pharmaceutical companies. There are more prescription drug options available to Americans than can be found anywhere else on the planet. As established previously in this chapter, we Americans spend more on drugs than people of any other country in the industrialized world. Therefore, if America, by comparison, has more and better conventional drugs, and we are using them more, we should have less of a cancer problem than any other country. Yet, as indicated earlier, Americans live fewer healthy years and have a cancer mortality rate as high as citizens of most other major countries. So, once again, the questions that are not being widely raised need to be. What are we doing wrong in the long, protracted war against cancer? Why isn't something working? What can we do better? What needs changing in our strategy? What are some alternatives? Isn't it past time for some unconventional thinking?

Marketing Trumps Research

Major Pharmaceutical companies spend an average of one-third of their total sales on marketing and promotion. The industry invests twice as much in marketing as it does on research and development. Table 10-2 shows almost $100 billion spent on marketing by ten major companies while only about half of that much went to research and development (Public Integrity 2008).

Table 10-2 Major Pharmaceutical Companies Marketing vs. R & D Spending (Billions)

Company	Marketing Cost	Research & Development
Pfizer	$16.9	$7.7
Johnson & Johnson	$15.9	$5.2
GlaxoSmithKline	$12.9	$5.2
Novartis	$8.9	$4.2
AstraZeneca	$7.8	$3.8
Merck & Co.	$7.4	$4.0
Roche	$7.2	$4.0
Bristol-Myers Squibb	$6.4	$2.5
Wyeth	$5.8	$2.5
Sanofi-Aventis	$5.6	$9.3
TOTAL	$94.8	$48.4

If the drugs produced by these corporations were having the positive results claimed, physicians and medical institutions would not need to be convinced by marketing campaigns costing billions of dollars. The exorbitant costs of cancer treatment drugs are related more to promoting the drugs to the oncologists than to the research and development of the drugs themselves.

Pharmaceutical executives would argue that it takes this level of marketing expenditures to differentiate their products from those of other companies. They would say that the high stakes business of big pharma necessitates the multi-billion dollar marketing expenses in order to stay competitive. However, in reality, the cartel-like nature of the industry allows it to function somewhat like the utility industries. Companies can agree to stake out segments of the market where they perform best and claim virtually exclusive rights to those segments. There is just enough competition in each segment to keep it from becoming monopolistic. In effect, that is how pharmaceutical companies operate.

In my opinion, the reason that big pharma spends so much on marketing is to make the stakes too high for the smaller entrepreneurial producer. Then, the medical practitioners, institutions, and patients see and hear little other than mainstream options for solutions to health issues. The institutional messages to oncologists, cancer researchers, and cancer patients are designed to be clear, compelling, and continuous. The messages convince all concerned that the answer to cancer is promulgation of more and better chemical formulas.

The drug industry is enormous and has evolved from the industrial giants of the world. Its control of its market and its favor from government have virtually excluded any outsider competition.

In Bed with the Fed

The conventional drug manufacturers and marketers enjoy the freedoms of high pricing and limited competition mostly because of the lack of government interference. Again, I am laissez-faire in my business philosophically. I believe the economy runs most efficiently with the least amount of government interference. But, in this case, the government's hands-off position is rather skewed in favor of the pharmaceutical industry to the detriment of entrepreneurial medicine. There is reluctance in Washington, D.C., to question the research and marketing strategies of big pharma. Tax breaks, protected markets, and generous fiscal policies seem to be free flowing to the big name pharmaceuticals from Congress and governmental agencies. Conversely, producers and researchers of natural, non-pharmacological options are not only excluded from the same favors, but are often blocked out of the competition through legislative constraints or enforcement of unnecessary rules. This is done within the pretense of public safety while big pharma thrives in the status quo of an imbalanced business environment.

A recent Center for Public Integrity investigation found that giant pharmaceutical companies spend over $100 million a year in federal lobbying and campaign donations. This is the largest lobbying expenditure of any industry in the nation. No other industry spends more money to sway public policy (Public Integrity 2008). The medicine makers employ the services of about 3,000 lobbyists at the federal level. Over a thousand of these are former federal officials who have valuable connections in the Congress, the FDA, the Department of Health and Human Services, and various other health-related offices. Seventy-five of the pharmaceutical lobbyists at the time of this writing are former members of Congress.

In addition to lobbying efforts, the industry is contributing to the political campaigns of unprecedented numbers of federal and state politicians. According to a recent survey by the Center for Responsive Politics, employees and political action committees within the pharmaceutical industry gave $133 million over a six-year period to the campaigns of candidates running for federal and state offices. Most of these contributions flowed through the "soft money" gray area within federal and state campaign finance laws (Public Integrity 2008). Most recipients were congressional members who sit on committees that decide on pharmaceutical issues.

Lobbying and campaign contributions are not the only ways the pharmaceutical industry influences congressional actions. The Center for Public Integrity reports that, during a 5 ½-year period from early 2000 to mid 2005, lawmakers and staffers accepted at least 325 free trips valued at over $600,000 from pharmaceutical companies or trade groups. This perk for congressional offices seems to be on the rise. In 2000, the drug industry spent $53,000 on these trips. That figure increased each year peaking at $181,000 at the end of the Center's report period. Typically, the number of these trips surges just prior to votes on significant legislation that has a major impact on the industry (Public Integrity 2008).

This massive lobbying and contribution effort certainly bears fruit. The U.S. government contributes more money to the development of new drugs in the form of tax breaks and subsidies than any other national government (Public Integrity 2008). The industry's two trade groups, PhRMA and the Biotechnology Industry Organization disclosed lobbying Congress on more than 1,600 bills over a recent six-year period. By the way, these two lobbyist groups are headed by two influential former members of Congress. Both of the former congressmen were on committees that regulated drug companies, and they each had sponsored several bills related to the industry (Public Integrity 20008). The top pharmaceutical corporations maintain a perpetual network that makes sure they will thrive in the highly profitable prescription drug market for decades to come. This is critically important to their survival. A market that would become more open to new integrative products and less protective of price levels would probably be the beginning of the end of the big pharma era as we know it.

Wanted: A New Political Paradigm

Before we get too laden with bias against big pharma, let's pause momentarily for a reality check. Would we like to see the huge pharmacy corporations completely fade away? No. The massive amount of capital in the industry ensures that we benefit from the most progressive research and development in the world. Our society can afford the finest health facilities and the most professional brain trust of medical experts available anywhere. Each of us benefits, probably daily, from the utmost in drugs, materials, and equipment. These "necessities" would not be there for us without the development, production, and distribution advantages of the monolith industry. We have paid dearly for such advantages. America's health culture includes continuous and aggressive pursuit of new and better products and services for our infirmities. Although we complain about the prices, we are apparently willing to pay them. Big pharma depends on our demand, and we depend on big pharma's supply.

Then, what is wrong? Let's review the problem. The problem is that relatively little effort is being made toward potential medical breakthroughs outside the realm of exclusive traditional, conventional medicine. Exploration of natural, non-pharmacological, non-toxic approaches to healing is suppressed by political actions from the industry and the government. The existence of big pharma is not the issue. The issue is that very promising enhancements to big pharma are not often allowed a place at the health care table. There is room for co-existence of integrative medicine with conventional medicine. The former complements the latter. That would be the best of all worlds. Let natural medicine compete to be included with conventional medicine in an open, free market. What a novel idea! Almost sounds like the principle the American economy was founded on.

The role of the government, in this case, should be to protect its citizens from harmful drugs and unqualified medical practitioners. In attempting to assume this role, the government has extended its authority far beyond protecting to the point of denying public access to reasonably safe natural medicines and practices. By reasonably safe, I am referring to products and practices that have not been proven adverse to use by humans, have every reason to be considered safe, and have proven in genuine scientific tests to be effective against various health problems. As I established previously, approved prescription drugs have proven to be adverse to human use and even deadly in many cases. If the same criteria were applied by the government and its health agencies to both conventional and natural products and practices equally, both would be made equally available to the open market. The bias that allows energetic research and testing of conventional proposals while non-pharmacological proposals sit on the sidelines is largely due to the political nature and culture of the entire medical community. The momentum of conventional medicine is fueled by (1) big pharma's dominance of the medical system, (2) the legislature and government agencies influenced by the largest lobbying effort in the country, and (3) the American tendency for acquiescence to the medical establishment.

A major political paradigm shift is critical to winning the cancer war. Congress, the FDA, the AMA, the NIH/NCI, the ACS, as well as prominent cancer centers and medical schools must accept natural, non-pharmacological cancer treatment options. They must be convinced that these options are a necessary and integral part of the overall war strategy. They need to take a hard, honest look at the lack of progress in our ability to overcome the disease over the past several decades. Such a shift would begin with the medical establishment acknowledging the slow progress of the last half-century and that headway could be gained by looking beyond the traditional, conventional treatment options. They would have to worry less about money and corporate survival and more about healing and a potential cure. Even though research and development of most unconventional proposals could not be market priced to generate a lucrative return on investment, certified laboratories should conduct the testing anyway supported by grants. The testing would have to be absolutely unbiased under the strictest of controls. Some of the arguably unnecessary restrictions on the clinical trials would have to be relaxed to accept a certain level of risk.

The risk factor is the principal claim that prohibits the testing and approving of prospective natural solutions. However, there is considerable risk in the testing and approval process for conventional options as well. How often are we subjected to the touting of the latest in conventional miracle drug or treatment just to learn in a few weeks or months that it believed to cause great harm and is being recalled? How many more years are we going to accept 1500 cancer deaths a day because experimenting with a complementary treatment option might possibly cause a few deaths or complications? We don't know the level of risk with much of any unconventional treatment options, because the government and the medical establishment will not permit the necessary clinical trials to even be initiated.

Every year, complementary cancer treatment prospects with great potential of success never get to the laboratory because of political opposition from government and industry or because the small return on investment generates too little incentive. Too much money is available to fund the status quo and too little money is available to make other options profitable. In either case, the solution is to somehow, some way, change the money equation. Laws must be passed to legislate the ethical high road, and money must be generated for testing of treatment alternatives. Both must happen.

A Political Model

There could and should be a best of both worlds. In fact, there should be just one world of cancer treatment products and practice with room for all options. That world ought to be characterized as inviting to the full spectrum of ideas and strategies employable against the disease. Laws should be enacted that place reasonable controls on the levels of contributions and other influences that the pharmaceutical industry lavishes on Congress and applicable government agencies. The government should restrict only the use of products and practices that have proven to be harmful rather than approving only those that meet often arbitrary standards. Let the doctor and patient decide, to a great extent, what is effective. Physicians need to be trained in all aspects of treatment, not just conventional, and be encouraged to prescribe, from among tested and approved options, what they think is best. Medical schools and medical centers should receive government incentive and private assistance to research and test natural treatment products and practices.

It goes against the grain of my nature to suggest increased government intervention into any area of the business environment. Generally, less government involvement in commerce results in a healthier economy. However, if the cartel attributes of big pharma are not contained, unconventional treatment options will never have a chance to be seriously considered. This would not be unduly restricting big pharma's access to government, but rather restoring government's freedom from the undue influence of big pharma. Only with the reduction of the hundreds of millions of dollars in drug industry influence will the government be inclined to give appropriate attention to possibilities from outside of the biggest corporations. Even if this monopolistic influence buying is reduced considerably, natural treatment proponents must ratchet up their government influence activities if they want a place at the table. A certain amount of lobbying effort is necessary to keep the government informed and updated. It will be a cost of doing business if integrative treatment is to mature. Congress and government health agencies should police themselves with the aid of all treatment proponents to maintain a balanced view of cancer treatment options.

A well informed, non-biased Congress should ensure that all cancer treatment options, conventional and unconventional, have the opportunity to prove themselves in fair clinical trials and free market competition. The only criteria for restrictions on testing, marketing, and use should be harmful effects that are not offset by the relief and healing ultimately produced. This determination of harmful effects should be made by a consensus of conventional and unconventional medicine practitioners. A preponderance of anecdotal and early clinical trial evidence showing exceptional promise and minimal risk should be sufficient grounds for initial approval of field application.

The development process for new drugs is broken and must be fixed. A recent study estimates the average cost of developing a new drug is over $800 million, and it takes an average of 12 years to get it to the market (Biopharmaceutical Research 2009). A fierce war against cancer cannot be waged with that kind of supply system. We are literally killing ourselves by accepting such a slow and burdensome process.

Imagine a field general reporting to the Department of Defense that he was losing the war, and being told to hang in there for 12 more years while they try to develop a better weapon. And, that is if they can find the $800 million to do the testing. That would be even more troubling to the general if he knew that many new weapons that might bring victory were available, but just hadn't passed the 12 years of study and testing yet. If a cure for cancer were introduced today, and even if it were a natural, available, non-toxic substance, almost seven million more victims would die before we could get the cure through our development process! How unacceptable is that? Even then, the likelihood is that it would be rejected in the process if it were not introduced through the conventional, big pharma industry. It is the FDA and the AMA, in partnership with the NCI, that manage our drug development system with the support of Congress. Laws should limit the ability of these agencies to overrule patients' freedom. Cancer victims deserve the right to choose natural products and practices expeditiously, as long as they are adequately tested to indicate little risk of harm and a reasonable potential of benefit.

Natural medicine and methodologies should be integrated into the curriculums of all medical schools. Medical Doctor degrees should require core courses in complements to conventional medicine. It is especially critical that oncologists have full knowledge of the myriad of non-toxic, non-invasive treatments that can be openly discussed and prescribed for patients that choose that direction. They need to be keenly aware of the latest in integrative treatment options and follow closely the research being conducted for such treatment. This has to be done in parallel with the opening up of the integrative medicine market and the lifting of the restrictions on its application. There is no advantage in open-minded doctors with constraints on their practice. Neither is there advantage in unconstrained practice with doctors ignorant of integrative medicine.

Medical schools have no incentive to add integrative medicine to their core curriculum. That incentive must come from the government and professional agencies. The Congress needs to enact legislation that legitimizes integrative medicine by mandating its inclusion in all medical schools. The AMA policies would have to change to encourage research and development of unconventional medicine with the same priority as conventional medicine. Results would be published in the journals and would be studied in the schools. Big pharma will probably never invest in research of alternatives to high-priced drugs because of poor return on investment. The obvious opportunity for such research would be within the major medical schools and medical centers. Their funding is primarily through government appropriations and private grants. Therefore, the future of integrative cancer treatment is in government funding earmarked for its research and development as well as private donors and foundations shifting their priorities toward the same purpose. Key government leaders would have to muster the courage to lead the charge in a sweeping change in the cancer war strategy. Major cancer foundations would have to change their objectives and priorities to support integrative treatment research as well as conventional research. How about a Race for the *natural* Cure?

This is what the "apolitical" war would look like with everyone focused on winning. The strategy would be clear with unified support. The federal and state governments would give equable support to all weapons and tactics necessary for victory. Professional support agencies in coordination with industrial suppliers would ensure the development and production of the best weapons without political bias or profiteering. Free market competition would assure the employment of the most efficient and effective weapons and operators. Field generals and battlefield commanders in the cancer war would be free to choose the weapons and tactics they deemed best. Troops on the front line could use a wide array of weapons and tactics depending on the enemy capability and movement. Unconventional forces and non-traditional methods of battle would catch the enemy off guard and keep them on the defensive. Ultimately, the lean, mean fighting machine would be victorious. It would have never tasted victory under its previous constraints and status quo.

Generally, two types of political approaches have characterized the wars of the past century. In WWI and WWII, political influences were directed almost entirely to uncompromising victory. How we won was less important than the determination to win. The victory over the European Axis was through the overwhelming employment of conventional forces. The victory over Japan was through the ultimate in unconventional force—the atomic bomb. Total victory in WWII was through the integration of conventional and unconventional weaponry. Although conventional forces were holding on in the Pacific, it took something fierce and previously unknown to bring Japan to a declaration of surrender. On the other hand, the Korea, Vietnam, Iraq, and Afghanistan wars were replete with political complexity. Winning was not as important as how we would win. The troops and their commanders were under countless constraints while Washington debated political ramifications. The nation's industries were not on a wartime footing, but essentially doing business as usual. The American citizens were much less committed to victory than they were in the World Wars. Compare the results.

Today, our arch enemy is not a nation. It is terrorism carried out by radical fundamentalists. Like cancer, this enemy doesn't identify itself until it is too late. Then, it goes into hiding among the normal, noncombatant population. Conventional warfare is virtually useless against it. Yet, that is in large measure what we are fighting it with. Terrorism can only be defeated by unconventional means, much of which may not have even been discovered or invented yet.

The war on cancer will only be won with the political and cultural resolve of the World Wars including their use of the unconventional. We cannot continue to fight it the way we fought our more recent wars—through politics.

CHAPTER 11

THE INSURANCE FACTOR

The availability of health insurance is a relatively recent factor in public health consumer decision making. Insurance policies for hospital care and other medical expenses were not introduced until after World War I. Less than a half century later, over 75% of all Americans had some form of health care coverage. As of 2009, at least 85% of Americans were covered, and, as evident in the recent health care reform, health insurance is now generally considered as an entitlement right by our society (U. S. News 2009). The first year of President Obama's presidency was virtually consumed with obtaining universal, full coverage health insurance for everyone in the country.

This exponential growth of the health insurance industry is both caused by and the cause of rising health care costs. It is both a necessity and a cost escalator. The costs of medical care in the early 20th century were so low that about the only insurance purchased was "sickness" insurance to provide income replacement in case of illness. As the century progressed, rising incomes along with advances in medical technology encouraged people to visit physicians more and accept more hospital stays. A new era of dependence on scientific medicine and new standards of licensure and care led to significantly increased costs to the patient. Medical school consolidation to control rising costs of educating physicians and stricter student entrance requirements put additional pressure on the supply, and thus the costs, of physicians' services.

The high demand and high cost of health care forced the creation of prepaid hospitalization plans which eventually became premium payment insurance plans. Blue Cross was the non-profit, mutual company that initially provided almost all of such hospital coverage. Although slow to adopt similar coverage, physicians eventually accepted the Blue Cross coverage for their services with the assistance of the AMA. By mid-century, the growth of the health insurance market became inviting to commercial insurance companies. Previously, the problem of adverse selection had discouraged other companies from entering the market. Adverse selection assumes that only those who are unhealthy or high risk will buy insurance, and there will be too few healthy people paying premiums to offset the costs of claims. Blue Cross had overcome adverse selection with the group insurance concept which required all members of insured groups, including employees of businesses, to be insured. This concept blew the market wide open to competition and made health insurance an expected employment benefit of workplaces across the nation. In the mid-60s, government sponsored Medicare and Medicaid closed the health insurance gap for the elderly and the poor making health care available and affordable for the large majority of the population.

Health insurance is a third-party payer which basically excludes the health care provider and beneficiary from the economic laws of supply and demand. As a third-party payer, the insurer eliminates the economic self-regulating exchange that would normally take place between the insured and the medical provider. Charges for physician services become less of a concern for both the patient and the doctor. Since the doctors are being paid by the insurance companies rather than the patients, they tend to charge higher rates for covered services. Since the bills are not being paid directly by the patients, they tend to choose more frequent and more sophisticated care. The same is true of the patient and hospital interchange. Now, I realize this is very fundamental economics and does not consider regulatory constraints, insurance deductibles, co-payments, etc. Nevertheless, the basic premise holds true. Medical costs have spiraled upward due, in large measure, to widely available health insurance.

The health care industry and the health insurance industry grew exponentially and in parallel during the 20th century, both directly supporting each other. This interdependence has had both a positive and a negative impact on all of us who require and support their services. On the positive side, the growth has allowed us to generally access and afford the best medical care known to mankind. On the negative side, costs of that medical care have escalated far beyond the consumer price index rate of growth. Spiraling medical costs have been largely caused by third-party payments from health insurance which circumvent normal supply and demand restraints. In other words, people have demanded more health care than they could have afforded without insurance, which has pushed health care prices upward. Although, this has been a privilege for our society from a health perspective, it causes health care cost inflation that keeps prices of both the care and the insurance out of reach for some. Since the two industries are interdependent, their connectivity ensures mutual agreement on almost any issue.

Therefore, the reluctance of the medical establishment to accept most CAM therapies prompts most insurance companies to deny claims for the same. Such insurance restrictions provide the medical practitioners the incentive to advise against CAM therapies. Patients then opt out of CAM therapies on the advice of their doctors and due to their own lack of insurance coverage. This is a continuous circle of frustration for proponents of integrative medicine.

The State of Insurance Coverage of Integrative Therapies

The premise of health insurance being both caused by and the cause of high medical care costs is the backdrop for what will be an abbreviated look at insurance and the new strategy. If more complementary therapies were available for more integrative oncologists, the overall costs of cancer treatment would likely be reduced. Presumably, the synergistic effect of complementary therapies in conjunction with conventional treatment would mean fewer treatments and more effective treatments. Therefore, less money would be spent on the most expensive drugs. Likewise, with more awareness and availability of integrative treatment, cancer patients would explore more treatment options with their oncologist resulting in probable cost savings. Such doctor–patient interaction in a CAM-sensitive environment would mean smaller health insurance claims. Smaller claims would result in smaller premiums. Obviously, the principal barrier to this vision is the reluctance of most oncologists to prescribe or provide referrals for complementary therapies. The next barrier is the reluctance of the health insurance companies to accept claims for most complementary therapies.

As noted in Chapter 1, over a third of American adults use some form of CAM. Some of this use is in coordination with a medical doctor, but most is not. Again, hardly any use of CAM is covered by insurance including Medicare and Medicaid. The justification for not covering treatment provided without the oversight of a medical doctor is understandable. Insurance companies reason that, in the absence of strict oversight by licensed and trained physicians, they are not able to distinguish legitimate treatments from "quackery." However, disallowing CAM treatments by, or under the supervision of, licensed and trained physicians cannot continue if integrative cancer treatment is to flourish under a new strategy.

The last few years have brought on a modest relaxation of insurance restrictions on selective CAM practices. Some insurance companies, for instance, have recently begun to provide varying degrees of coverage for chiropractic treatment and acupuncture. Acupuncturist coverage is even mandated in California, Florida, Maine, Montana, New Mexico, Nevada, Oregon, Rhode Island, Texas, Virginia, and Washington. Massage therapy is covered by law in Maryland, New Hampshire, Utah, and Washington. Naturopath coverage is mandated in Alaska, Montana, Vermont, and Washington (Insure.com 2009).

Chiropractic

Individual states have considerable control over what insurance companies will or will not cover. Some states mandate limited coverage for chiropractic treatment in all health insurance plans. In these states, most insurance companies place limitations on the number of treatments covered and the amount of payment for each treatment. Some plans limit covered treatment to spinal manipulation only to avoid paying for massage treatments, ultrasound treatments, etc. Another restriction often included is covering only those treatments obtained through a network of participating contract chiropractors.

Medicare will cover only manual manipulation of the spine. The Social Security Act defines chiropractor as a physician for only one service, subluxation of the spine. Chiropractic coverage is optional under Medicaid, so each state determines whether to provide coverage. Most states limit Medicaid payments in the same manner as Medicare.

Acupuncture

Acupuncture has more recently entered the coverage list of some insurance companies. Like chiropractic, plans will usually limit their coverage to treatments provided by a licensed MD or DO (Doctor of Osteopathy). Some companies will cover procedures by state licensed acupuncturists, but only when recommended or referred by a licensed medical doctor. Medicare specifically excludes acupuncture treatments. Those few states that provide coverage under their Medicaid program limit the benefits or restrict coverage to treatments in a hospital or doctor's office.

Other Treatments

Insurance rarely covers any other types of CAM treatments except in those states with certain mandatory coverage. Most plans include phrases like, "Coverage only for services provided by a legally licensed physician performing within the scope of their license." This allows the companies to refuse coverage of treatments they determine to be too far removed from "Western" or traditional medicine.

Herbal medications, homeopathic treatments, nutritional supplements, and other treatments within the category of holistic medicine are rarely, if ever, covered by health insurance. Almost all plans require covered medications to be available by prescription only and FDA approved, thereby paying for nothing obtained "over-the-counter."

Occasionally, there is some flexibility in coverage of CAM if a licensed medical provider prescribes and offers the medication or procedure directly as part of an office visit. In these cases, the medication or procedure is considered inclusive of the office visit. For cancer patients, this might include natural supplements, massage therapy, acupuncture, chelation, etc. during an office visit.

Supplemental Insurance Options

If individuals want insurance coverage for CAM treatments, about the only option is to pay extra for some type of supplemental coverage or medical savings plan. It is ironic that, if you desire a complementary treatment that is low cost and, in all likelihood, reduces the total cost of conventional treatment, you have to pay more for the extra insurance coverage.

A few insurance companies offer a CAM rider, or supplemental coverage, for a considerably higher premium and usually a higher deductible. Some plans, particularly health maintenance organizations (HMO's) that use contracted providers, may cover certain CAM treatments offered at deep discounts by the providers. A small number of insurance companies will write a CAM treatment policy separate from any other policy, but, again, almost always with significantly higher premiums and deductibles.

Some employers offer Medical Savings Accounts or Health Savings Accounts. These are tax sheltered savings accounts that can be drawn on to pay for medical treatments and supplies that are not covered by insurance. However, the accounts can only be used for charges that are considered tax deductible by the Internal Revenue Service. Fortunately, these include some CAM treatments performed by physicians, surgeons, specialists, and other medical practitioners. The IRS does not recognize any medicines other than prescription.

The Typical Situation of the Insured

Let's take a look at a hypothetical, but realistic, scenario of a cancer patient who desires integrative therapy. We will call our patient, Brad.

Brad was diagnosed with cancer and immediately referred to a surgeon for removal of a tumor. After the operation, the surgeon and Brad's family doctor recommended a few oncologists in the area. His previous general knowledge of cancer and his intense study since the diagnosis had convinced him to seek an experienced integrative oncologist. The oncologists his doctor recommended all turned out to have no experience in or desire to practice integrative oncology. Finding an oncologist or even a cancer clinic that offers CAM treatments became a challenge for Brad. He and his wife searched the internet, looked in the yellow pages, phoned local clinics, and contacted friends and relatives looking for any information about integrative treatment availability. The only clinic in the local area that fit his criteria limited CAM use to acupuncture, massage, and other pain management therapies. He could travel some distance to reputable clinics where he could get expert counsel and care in several CAM options that complemented chemotherapy and radiation therapy.

Brad, with the support of his family and friends, decided to accept the travel inconvenience and avail himself of several integrative options designed for his particular needs. The next big hurdle was how to pay for it. He had an excellent health insurance plan through his work with even a catastrophic provision for serious diseases. Even so, each of the clinics advised him to obtain preauthorization from his insurance company and offered to assist in that process. The insurance company quickly responded that, after a $500 annual deductible, they would pay 80% of all qualifying hospital and physician charges as well as approved conventional therapy. They cautioned, though, that claims for complementary therapies offered by these clinics would be considered on a case-by-case basis. They indicated that most would be denied and would become the responsibility of the insured.

Therefore, only the chemotherapy, radiation therapy, and any further surgery that Brad received would likely be reimbursed, and then only at 80%. He had a small supplemental policy with limitations that would not pay nearly all of the out-of-pocket 20% and, again, little or nothing toward complementary therapies. Facing six-figure charges for at least several weeks of therapy, he calculated an anticipated after-insurance personal financial obligation that almost matched his home mortgage balance. Even if he settled for conventional treatment alone resulting in total remission, he would trade his health crisis for a financial crisis.

If he wished to take advantage of the clinically proven complementary therapies prescribed by his integrative oncologist, he would have to pay almost every dollar of those therapies out of his own pocket. Meticulous coordination with the medical records and billing departments might result in a few specific complementary therapies being recognized by the insurance company as covered treatment. But, his costs for the vast majority of the prescribed, but non-covered, therapies would be unaffordable, especially when added to the out-of-pocket charges for the conventional therapies.

Brad had an agonizing decision to make in consultation with his family, his prospective oncologist, his financial advisor, and his accountant. Such a huge financial decision should not face a person just diagnosed with cancer. Every legitimate medical advantage possible should be on the table for a cancer patient's choosing without regard to the bureaucratic policies of health insurance providers. All therapies that are legal, proven effective, and available at reasonable cost should qualify for insurance coverage. Evidence-based complementary therapies that have great potential for expediting healing and reducing side effects should be covered as fully in insurance plans as conventional therapies.

A Personal Note:

After three years of chemotherapy, radiation, and surgery, Connie's total treatment costs had exceeded $500,000. I was blessed with a good, caring primary health insurance provider and an equally good supplemental plan. Had I been uninsured or minimally insured, I would probably have been facing bankruptcy. However, as indicated previously, after exhausting the capabilities of conventional treatment, we traveled to Mexico for an integrative treatment protocol, much of which was evidence-based and available in the U.S. through licensed physicians. The reason we went to Mexico was to access a few therapies that were not available in the U.S. Our insurance company advised us in advance that none of the $10,000 worth of these CAM therapies would be paid.

I strongly encourage all readers to review their insurance coverage and confirm that there are sufficient benefits to cover prolonged cancer treatment for each family member. Then, think through whether you would seek complementary therapies and, if so, how you would pay for it. Until we progress to a new strategy, a financial plan for cancer is essential. Remember, there is about a one in three chance that you and members of your family will be diagnosed with it sooner or later. That means there is over a 60% probability that either you or your spouse will have cancer and will incur the financial challenges that it brings.

The Irony of It All

It seems rather absurd that the insurance industry will not agree to pay for a legitimate treatment that costs much less than the treatment they are more than willing to cover. Scientific studies have confirmed the ability of many complementary therapies to enable the patient to tolerate the conventional treatments better and, therefore, to enhance the effectiveness of the treatments. Some complementary therapies act as a booster to conventional treatments allowing them to have more impact with less toxicity and in fewer applications. When these lower cost therapies can increase the efficacy and decrease the dosage and/or duration of higher cost conventional treatment, the health provider wins, the insurance company wins, and, most importantly, the patient wins!

As long as all health insurance companies have comparable policies on allowable benefits, there is little incentive for any of them to change. The 60% of the insured population whose insurance is employment based will generally oppose change. Changing plans is inconvenient for the insured, causes them to suspect fewer benefits, and may not personally save them much, if any, since the employer may pay all or much of the premium. So, the status quo is unfortunately a convenient option for both the insurer and the insured even though premium and claims savings could be realized by both if scientifically proven complementary therapies were covered.

One solution to this dilemma would be for a few insurance companies to break away from the pack and offer the same coverage for complementary therapies that they offer for conventional therapies. This would be a bold move because there is hardly any precedent for valuation of complementary therapies. Claim payments for complementary physician services, equipment usage, and prescriptions would have to be standardized, at least within geographical regions. Limits on frequency, range, and duration of treatments would have to be established. New and precise definitions of treatments would have to be agreed on between medical providers and insurance companies. Restrictive benefits language would have to be carefully crafted to clearly draw the line between evidenced based complementary therapy and unproven alternative therapy.

The outcome of this industry-reshaping venture would be a quantifiable reduction in cancer treatment claim levels for the participating insurer. Reduced claim expenditures would eventually translate to reduced premium payments. Promotional efforts of the insurers would emphasize their integrative treatment coverage and lower premiums bringing them a wave of additional applications. I believe such an initiative by a few leading visionary insurers would pay dividends that would draw other companies into the new concept. It would pave the way to a new cooperative paradigm between the insurance industry and integrative oncology.

An Essential Strategy Element

Health insurance has become a basic necessity of life in our modern times. It would be a challenge for most people to pay for their routine medical care and extremely difficult for them to pay for extended illnesses, chronic diseases, and major accidents. Very few individual or family financial crises would be more crippling than paying out-of-pocket for the average series of cancer treatments. Dr. Allen Lichter of the American Society of Clinical Oncology said that sticker shock is hitting cancer patients hard, especially those without health insurance. For instance, new and more advanced biotech drugs have led to treatment rounds costing $100,000 or more. Dr. Lichter noted that the cost of cancer care is rising 15 percent per year.

Even with good, but non-supplemented, health insurance coverage, one in five people diagnosed with cancer use all or most of their savings for the extensive medical costs. Those with no insurance or insufficient insurance have higher medical costs (hospitals and physicians usually charge more for services not covered by insurance), poorer outcomes, and higher rates of death. Such services to the uninsured are either paid by Medicaid (ultimately the taxpayers) or written off by the hospitals and providers. Provider write-offs, of course, are ultimately recovered in increased charges to the insured which, again, places upward pressure on overall therapy costs. Some level of cost relief for the uninsured and underinsured would be realized by greater use of complementary therapies. These lesser costs would mean less recovery costs passed on by providers to the insured. All cancer patients deserve the option of integrative treatments without agonizing over insurance coverage. The new strategy for the war on cancer can never be fully realized without an industry-wide acceptance of complementary therapy insurance claims

A Challenge to the Health Insurance Industry

A precedent was set a few years ago for health insurance coverage of CAM therapies. Several years of research resulted in finding that lifestyle changes in diet, exercise, vitamin supplements, and spiritual focus could reverse coronary heart disease. Medicare analysis subsequently revealed that adding these CAM therapies to their normal coverage for bypass surgeries and drug therapies would save them an average claims payout of almost $30,000 per heart patient. Other insurance companies followed suit (Ornish 2005). It would only be a small step to analyze similar savings on cancer therapies.

In 2008, direct medical costs of all cancer health expenditures in America was $93 billion (ACS 2009). No wonder cancer benefits are a hot topic among health insurance companies. With cancer-related claims approaching $100 billion, insurance companies are obviously looking for ways to reduce the costs of cancer therapies. They would do well to join in the exploration of options to cover CAM therapies as cost saving complements to conventional therapies.

The recent health care reform debate that consumed America had many facets. Regrettably, hardly a word was heard about integrative medicine in general and certainly not about integrative oncology. This was a missed opportunity to address the insurance for CAM treatment issue. We must not miss further opportunities.

CHAPTER 12

THE EDUCATION FACTOR

I have a friend whose son had just graduated from medical school and had begun his residency at the time of this writing. This young man, whom I have known since he was in elementary school, was always intelligent beyond his years, very dependable, and just an all around fine kid. I recently had a long discussion with him regarding exposure to integrative medicine during the educational journey to becoming a doctor.

He explained that undergraduate objectives of future medical school candidates involve completing the prerequisite courses for medical school, maintaining a high grad point average (GPA), and scoring high on the Medical College Admissions Test (MCAT). An undergraduate degree for a prospective doctor can be in almost any field of study from biology to music. However, all medical schools have similar prerequisite courses that must be completed and a GPA, particularly in those courses, that is highly competitive. These prerequisites also prepare the prospective medical school student for the MCAT. Medical schools do not require any CAM-related courses in undergraduate work. One might find some CAM-related courses in various departments of universities that include, for example, nutrition, meditation, mind-body therapy, or eastern culture medicine. But, this subject matter would not be required by a medical school, and the MCAT would not test such knowledge. Therefore, the likelihood that a premed student would be made formally aware of any aspect of integrative medicine is about zero.

When I asked my friend's son what, if any, exposure to integrative medicine he had received once he entered medical school, he indicated that there had been very little. His only connection to the practice of CAM during medical school came through a couple of lectures on the subject that were required, but with no accountability. His coursework, on occasion, emphasized the necessity for doctors to understand that their patients may be using CAM on their own and to coordinate their treatments accordingly. He and his peers were taught the characteristics of some unconventional options they might encounter with patients, but only for the purpose of avoiding potential adverse effects of combining those options with conventional medicine. There was virtually no required instruction to suggest that CAM should be integrated routinely with conventional practice.

After completing medical school, this new MD began his residency program in his chosen field. For him and other graduates, this included two or three more years of intense, supervised practice in a major hospital or university medical center. Here, again, the only prospect of participating in or even observing integrative medicine would be if the particular residence institution had a major CAM program. Even then, unless the new doctors made a special effort to align themselves with the practice of CAM, they would not gain much familiarity with it. With very few exceptions, medical doctors in America today complete their entire scholastic journey to certification in their desired field of practice with almost no exposure to CAM and with little concept of integrative medicine.

The small minority of physicians who are experienced in integrative medicine and who teach and advocate CAM as a vital part of their practice have almost all attained that advantage through experiences gained well after their formal education. Some have been drawn to the successes of integrative medicine though their interaction with colleagues. Others have become attuned to the evidence of CAM advantages from clinical trials. Still others have developed a passion for unconventional, yet evidence-based, medicine and are simply following their heart. Unfortunately, until or unless medical institutions of learning make integrative medicine a core aspect of their curriculum and training, its practice will continue to be relegated to the periphery of health care.

The Premier Universities

The most respected universities that prepare new physicians should take the lead in furthering the future of integrative medicine. Many of these iconic institutions have planted the seeds of CAM within their framework by establishing a separate center so named. This is a significant first step, but it is just that—a first step. Most of these centers are focused on health care services rather than on education. Very few of the schools have fully integrated the subject matter into their required curriculum for medical doctors.

When I was a college freshman, one of my professors required that his students subscribe to the *U.S. News and World Report* magazine and read it weekly for class discussion. He described it as the best and most unbiased reporting of relevant news and useful information. I have continued to enjoy its no-nonsense approach to journalism and especially its periodic "lists of the best" features. Each year, *U.S. News*, as it is commonly called, evaluates a series of institutions from public schools to hospitals to retirement communities, and more. Of course, I watch each year for the list of top medical schools.

The *U.S. News* "Best Medical Schools for 2009" list was divided into two categories of *Research* and *Primary Care*. The schools were then prioritized in each category based on rigid standards of an independent evaluation group. I have listed in Table 12-1 the top ten schools from both categories taking into account some overlap of schools between the categories. With the overlap, 19 schools were in the top 10 of one or both categorized listings. Since I am not in the business of further ranking specific schools in this book, I have listed them alphabetically. I have also added the integrative medicine programs and centers next to the schools that have established them.

Table 12-1   2009 Best Medical Schools (U.S. New & World Report)
and Their Integrative Medicine Programs or Centers

Medical School	Integrative Medicine Program/Center
Columbia University	The Rosenthal Center for CAM
Duke University	Duke Integrative Medicine
Harvard University	Osher Institute
Johns Hopkins University	Center for CAM
Michigan State University	
Oregon Health & Science University	Women's Primary Care/Integ. Med
Stanford University	Stanford Center for Integrative Med
University of California-Los Angeles	Collaborative Centers for Integ. Med
University of California-San Francisco	Osher Center for Integrative Med
University of Colorado-Denver	Center for Integrative Medicine
University of Iowa (Carver)	
University of Minnesota	Center for Spirituality and Healing
University of Massachusetts-Worcester	Center for Mindfullness
University of North Carolina-Chapel Hill	Program on Integrative Medicine
University of Pennsylvania	CAM at Penn
University of Vermont	Program in Integrative Medicine
University of Washington	UW Integrative Medicine Program
Washington University-St. Louis	
Yale University	Integrative Medicine Center-Griffin

These medical schools, rated by an independent agency, have varying levels of efforts going toward the advancement of integrative medicine. As illustrated, all but three of them have officially established an integrative medicine program or center connected with the school. The programs or centers provide a broad scope of CAM research and/or clinical practice. Those three without a CAM program or center may have varying degrees of specific CAM studies and activities going on, but are not widely engaged in the effort. Each of those schools with such a program or center also happens to be a member of the Consortium of Academic Health Centers for Integrative Medicine (CAHCIM). This advancement of integrative medicine by these schools is commendable, and we applaud them for their inclusion of integrative medicine in their educational and clinical objectives. However, the degree to which the schools actually prepare their students to pursue integrative medicine and CAM therapies is minimal.

As I looked into the curriculum of each of the top schools, I saw only one that required integrative medicine/CAM courses for medical doctor students. The University of California – San Francisco has established several courses relating to integrative medicine and CAM in its core curriculum. The University also offers numerous such courses as popular electives. That came as no surprise, since UCSF is the host for the Osher Center for Integrative Medicine, probably the major organization of its kind for coordinating the inclusion of integrative medicine into academic and clinical programs. The school is also very involved in the CAHCIM and provides an aggressive program of guest lecturers, special events, and opportunities for hands-on experience in integrative medicine.

Some other schools on the list have integrative medicine courses posted on their course curriculum as electives. I was disappointed to find, though, that some of these top schools offer absolutely no integrative medicine courses. Even a few of them that have the integrative medicine programs and centers and are members of CAHCIM have no apparent academic offerings for their students in those subjects. Most of the programs and centers are for clinical application, public information, and research with little or no involvement in the academic realm of their schools. Some schools schedule a few optional presentations and seminars on latest advances in CAM or offer rotations in CAM clinics, but have no credit courses available. Hence, even though there is obvious interest and activity in integrative medicine within these prominent institutions, most provide scant opportunity for their students to become skilled in its practice or to even to be formally introduced to it.So, how do medical students become familiar with and learn to practice integrative medicine and CAM therapies? Most of them don't. And, there lies the problem. Many medical students fresh out of premed don't know enough about integrative medicine to even consider it in their medical school application process. Unless a medical student has a personal penchant for integrative medicine, and therefore applies to a school that he or she knows to offer at least adequate electives in the subject, he or she will go into residency with hardly a clue about it. If they enter medical school and then develop an affinity for the practice, it will probably be too late, because their school will not likely offer anything on it.

I believe that hundreds more students would develop an interest in integrative medicine if they were exposed to it in medical school each year. For many, that interest would not be stirred up by influences outside of their academics, but would come through assigned studies. Required courses in integrative medicine would undoubtedly fill voids in hungry minds of many young physician candidates who would be searching for new and exciting approaches to their chosen professions.

We shouldn't even have to suggest ways to draw students' attention to integrative medicine. Truth is, integrative medicine should not even be viewed as something students need to be drawn to. It is not like a student's leaning toward family practice, specialized medicine, or surgery. Integrative medicine should be ubiquitous throughout all medical disciplines. It should be equivalent to studies in anatomy, immunology, and pathology—required core curriculum.

There are numerous categories of integrative medicine practice that are proven to be generally beneficial to the effectiveness of traditional medicine. Dietary programs to accompany cardiovascular remedies are an example. Within those categories, there are usually several methodologies that are specifically designed and clinically tested to complement certain other treatments for better results. For instance, specific foods eaten at particular intervals have been proven to reduce certain cancer treatment side effects. These disciplines should be a part of the medical student curriculum as surely as radiology and pharmacology.

The integration of CAM into every aspect of medical scholarship is essential to the preparation of doctors for the best future of medicine. It is critical to the new strategy that this integration begin in the most elite medical schools and proliferate through the entire system of education for medical professionals.

CHAPTER 13

THE EVIDENCE FACTOR

You may have watched *Living Proof*, a 2008 television movie starring Harry Connick, Jr. The film is based on the true story of Dr. Dennis Slamon who helped develop the breast cancer drug Herceptin. The screen play was adapted from the book, *HER-2: The Making of Herceptin, a Revolutionary Treatment for Breast Cancer*, by Robert Bazell. Dr. Slamon, played by Connick, was a research doctor who stayed constantly frustrated about the more than 8 years it took (1988 to 1996) to get the drug approved for use. He was convinced early on that the new drug was a breakthrough of major proportion that would revolutionize breast cancer treatment.

Dr. Slamon's first set back was the termination of funding by the pharmaceutical company for which he was developing the drug. The company got nervous about the lawsuits other companies had recently incurred with new cancer drugs during and after laboratory testing. Dr. Slamon had to shift to dependence on private funding which was difficult to come by. Hundreds of millions of dollars had to be raised to fund the extremely complex process. Several years of funding by the Revlon Foundation and numerous charity balls ultimately underwrote the work. Then, highly successful tests of the drug on laboratory animals were dismissed by the governing agencies as not being applicable to humans. Additionally, finding women for the clinical trials who met the constrained protocols proved to be a major undertaking. Sadly, some patients involved in the tests died, but Slamon's work eventually changed the course of breast cancer treatment. It went through three trials before gaining approval from the FDA.

This movie was a public indictment of the randomized control trial process that stifles medical innovation in cancer treatment. It exemplified the typical process of getting a potential life-saving medicine from concept to approval. The process is slow, complicated, politically sensitive, and extremely expensive. Dr. Slamon experienced delays from disinterest, competition, endless bureaucratic hurdles, legal challenges, and funding constraints. It affected his personal and professional life. Most other researchers would have given up long before the success that ultimately resulted from his dogged persistency. Fortunately, Herceptin is now a widely used drug that has saved or extended the lives of thousands of HER-2 breast cancer patients.

About one of four breast cancer patients have tumors that are characterized as HER-2. HER-2 stands for Human Epidermal growth factor Receptor 2. These tumors tend to grow and spread more quickly than other tumors. Herceptin is an antibody that attacks the HER-2 tumor specifically. Administered intravenously, the drug binds exclusively to the HER-2 receptor arresting the growth phase of the cancer cell. It suppresses angiogenesis (blood vessel generation for the cancer cell). It is generally used in combination with chemotherapy, but has hardly any of the chemotherapy side effects. The achievement of this drug maintains the hope that such targeted drugs will someday let patients skip harsher chemotherapy, radiation, and surgery along with all of their harmful effects. The discovery of Herceptin is certainly one of the success stories of modern cancer therapy. The down side of the story is that it took eight years and Herculean efforts to make it available to cancer sufferers. During those eight years, about 365,000 women were diagnosed with HER-2 breast cancer and could have benefited substantially by Herceptin.

The Agonizing Process

Recall from Chapter 10 that the average process of working one candidate product through the new-medicine approval system takes more than a decade and costs an average of over $800 million. Keep in mind that, during the typical drug testing process, over six million more people die of cancer. The following steps describe this process in very summarized and simplified form.

1. Discovery Laboratory.

A new medicine is determined to be potentially beneficial in tumor apoptosis (killing the cancer cells) or in blocking pathways of support to cancer cells. In-vitro and/or animal models may be established to demonstrate its efficacy. The substance must be screened for acceptable properties such as absorption, distribution, metabolism, elimination, and toxicology.

2. Preclinical Development.

If step one proves the substance worthy of additional testing, safety and toxicology studies must further prove its safe use in various animal experiments. In this phase, the medicine must also be fully characterized including molecular weight and structure as well as solubility. Comparisons of intake modalities will be made among oral liquid, tablet, capsule, and IV doses. A maximum tolerated dose will be established. The most successful formulation will be produced in a pilot clinical batch. Quality control testing of this clinical batch includes the determination of optimal temperatures and humidity levels. These environmental tests can take up to four years while other trial phases are underway. Should these tests show degradation or breakdown of the active ingredient, the entire trial can be delayed until the problem is resolved.

3. Investigational New Drug (IND) filing.

If the substance passes all of the preclinical testing, it is submitted to the appropriate regulatory agency for the IND filing. Here, the regulatory agency will investigate the previous testing through record reviews and inspections. This step is always subject to the agency's backlog of investigations and must be completed prior to the beginning of clinical trials.

4. Clinical Trials.

Clinical trials are a giant step into testing of the product's effect on humans. Volunteers are enlisted to participate in random control trials where they are randomly selected to receive either the medicine being tested or a placebo. In the testing of cancer products, the volunteers are usually those patients who have received and not responded to available therapies. Clinical trials are divided into four phases of testing.

Phase I. These are usually small trials to test the safety and optimal doses of the product in human volunteers. The safety and amounts that were determined from previous testing are confirmed applicable for humans through trial and error.

Phase II. Further safety investigation along with efficacy is tested in this phase. The volunteers are narrowed down to those who have the specific condition that the product is believed to treat. Strict parameters are set to ensure that trial results cannot be attributed to therapies external to those being tested. Certain previous medical care or self-medication may be deemed as disqualifications from this trial phase. Vital physical data is collected from participating patients frequently to include blood pressure, pulse, pain levels, mobility, comfort, etc. Much of this data is sourced from blood samples, body eliminations, and questionnaires. This phase is somewhat lengthy in order to obtain a representative sampling over an extended period of product use.

Phase III. This third phase is initiated only if the first two phases are totally successful. It broadens the scale of investigation to multiple clinical sites and includes many more volunteers—often thousands. Again, considerable time and effort is expended here to observe, record, and analyze the wide-ranging effects of the product on a large population. If results are successful within strict parameters, the product developers apply to market it for use under the relatively narrow conditions of the testing process. Once approved for the market, the product is made available for medical providers and promoted accordingly.

Phase IV. If the manufacturer wishes to investigate further uses of the product or analyze post market efficacy and/or adverse events, this final phase is the optional opportunity to collect further data.

Obviously, this is a painstakingly slow process with much redundancy. Whether testing conventional drugs or integrative products, the time required for testing and the constraints of the testing greatly inhibit the development of new and promising products. For instance, curcumin discussed in Chapter 5 has been getting a lot of attention lately as a natural, non-toxic substance that appears to attack cancer cells without harming healthy cells. It has proven effective in animal experiments and is presently in early clinical trials. Even though this normal food item has shown no harmful side effects, it may take eight years or more to work it through the phases described above. To require that any natural medicine candidate be subjected to the same safety and tolerance process as a chemical based drug is an unnecessary delay in the clinical trial process. The inordinate amount of time to test any and all new cancer treatment possibilities must be a new strategy target.

How Much Evidence Is Enough?

For curcumin or any other natural treatment complement, the question is whether the full clinical trial system is absolutely necessary to obtain their approval. Must we necessarily know <u>how</u> it works, or is it enough to know <u>that</u> it works? Two things are paramount in determining whether the use of a medicine is ethically and morally right or wrong: (1) is it safe and (2) is it effective. If it is not safe, prescribing it violates basic societal principles and law as well as the Hippocratic Oath. If it is not effective, prescribing it is a scam and a crime. But, how should we define safety and effectiveness relative to the potential for less human suffering and extended human life?

After a product or procedure has passed the rigorous safety tests on humans in phase I, should patients whose condition it has the likelihood of treating effectively be denied it? Should it not be available to them particularly if they are informed of risk levels and still volunteer to use it? Presently, if something has proven safe in the early phases of testing, and could possibly cure your cancer or extend your life, you must wait until it has been tested in large populations under almost all conditions before you can benefit from it. Unless you are among the lucky few who meet the narrow qualifications for the advanced randomized control trials, and you don't draw the placebo, you will likely never have the opportunity to benefit from it. I believe that, if patients could benefit significantly from a discovery that was deemed safe in a Phase I trial, they should have the option to sign a release and receive the treatment. To do otherwise should be a crime.

Shouldn't acceptable evidence include both modern scientific research and the experience of hundreds of years of practice? I submit that anecdotal, or testimonial, justification for the use of a product or procedure should be a consideration. Granted, anecdotal data alone should not be the sole basis for agency approval, but it should be a major factor. The term "anecdotal evidence" is not an oxymoron as most conventional researchers profess. Scientists can analyze anecdotes of how certain properties or behaviors have affected people with certain conditions over time. If enough people get the same results from a particular practice, it works! The evidence is not in the means; it is in the end— the person.

Obviously, no provider or patient wants to use medicine without evidence of efficacy. The question is what is acceptable evidence? The mantra of conventional medicine is "evidence-based practice." However, the new cancer strategy should also consider "practice-based evidence." There are many practices that have been effective for thousands of years but are not practiced today simply because medical science has "insufficient evidence" of their validity. They appear to have worked for the alchemists and the eastern medicine practitioners, but they just can't pass the modern laboratory test standards. Some of these practices can't make it to human testing because they can't even meet the pretrial criteria. Sometimes, perfect medicine can be the enemy of good medicine if the perfect is unattainable or too late.

Physical Science Criteria Are Not Always Valid for Medical Science

I participated in the recent Institute of Medicine Summit on Integrative Medicine and Health of the Public. In a breakout session, NIH researcher, Perry

Skeath, explained that the way we apply physical science standards of validity and control to medical research doesn't always work. Skeath is a second-career research transplant from physical science (medical device development) to medical science (patient care). From this combination, he has experienced two fundamentally different research domains of natural phenomena: (1) physical and (2) mental, or psychological. He talked about how different domains of natural phenomena need different research paradigms, yet that has not generally been accepted. In his previous work, his only valid data was what could be observed physically and quantified. Testing relied on randomization which, with enough observations, screened out certain variables. However, he found that medical science included psychological, emotional, and spiritual factors that could not necessarily be observed and quantified. There is much more to consider in medical science than just the physical phenomenon. Medical scientists must have a broader view of what constitutes nature and analyze qualitative as well as quantitative data.

According to Skeath, one could look at the tremendous success of the physical sciences and think that approach is the best approach to science that we know. It could be considered the gold standard for all sciences and applied as such. However, some methodologies, theories, and principles that lead to rapid progress and huge successes in one science may actually be a hindrance when applied to another science. For example, the principle that the only valid sources of data are those that can be observed physically, does not make sense for the psychological sciences. Consciousness, thoughts, and the mind, which are non-physical, need to be studied and treated subjectively in psychology.

The physical science testing criteria served the medical community well in the move from alchemy to evidence-based medicine. It served as the standard and the template for all medical experiments. But, like all progressive knowledge, as the practice of medicine matured, some assumptions didn't hold up. Medical scientists must have a broader view of what constitutes nature and analyze qualitative as well as quantitative data. All understanding of science and reality needs to be kept open to question and revision. This shift toward a better understanding of testing criteria is both the cause and the effect of the growing acceptance of integrative medicine. That shift has been slow partly due to lack of acceptable non-physical methodology and non-physical theory.

How are scientists to make progress in developing methodologies, theories, and practices appropriate for medical science when their education has taught them that many of those considerations are not regarded as scientifically valid? Perry Skeath's epiphany during his transition from the physical to the medical sciences is an example of what is needed across the gamut of medical research and practice, especially regarding oncology. We must be open to exploring new methodologies that our physics-based science rarely recognizes as existing. We must be just as concerned about a treatment's effect on a multiplicity of subjective considerations as well as its effect on the tumor cell.

The new strategy requires a new concept of medical research and testing and a rethinking of what constitutes safety and efficacy. Research must allow an acceptable level of subjectivity. Testing must be shortened in length and broadened in scope. Safety must be relative to criticality of need. And, efficacy must be determined by both physical and non-physical scientific evidence.

PART 4

THE NEW STRATEGY VISION

CHAPTER 14

THE FUTURE OF CANCER

The new war strategy proposed by this book is a better road to a destination. It is more efficient, more comfortable, safer, and faster. The new strategy is not a turn choice at an intersection. It is not an optional scenic route that winds through nature settings. It is not a detour that departs from the main thoroughfare. It is not an access road that parallels the expressway until you can get back on. It is, in fact, a new expressway that leads to the intended destination, but with many advantages.

The New Expressway

Have you ever traveled the same road for years, then one day you notice that a new highway is being built almost parallel to it that looks to be straighter, wider, and smoother? You watch with interest as construction progresses. Meanwhile, you continue along your same old route every day. Your traditional road is crooked, bumpy, slow, and has a history of accidents. Shoulders are non-existent, bridges are narrow, and signage is poor. You have celebrated patched pot holes, but the patches can't seem to keep up with the damages to the original asphalt. Finally, one day, you notice the barricades are gone at the entry to the new expressway, and a few drivers are gladly taking advantage of the opportunity to drive it.

Over the next few days, you observe a few more drivers opting for the new choice. Not convinced though, you and many other drivers are content to drive the old road. Why? Well, you are very familiar with the original road, and you haven't heard a lot about the new highway except from a few media sources. Almost everyone you know personally is still using the old road. You understand that the new expressway should get you to your destination faster, more safely, and more comfortably. But, what if you get on it and it's not all it's hyped up to be? The map still shows the old road, so how can you be sure where the expressway leads? Besides, you also hear that the old road is going to be resurfaced someday. Probably better stick with what you know than risk something new, at least until you learn more about the new way.

Any time we are faced with something new, we are hesitant to commit ourselves to it until we understand it and are convinced it is in our best interests. Hopefully, what you have learned so far in this book has helped you to understand the advantages of integrative medicine, particularly as it applies to integrative oncology. Moreover, I trust that you agree on the essentiality of integrative oncology in winning the war on cancer. In this chapter, I want to present a very optimistic vision of the march to victory in this war. A vision should be something almost beyond comprehension—virtually unreachable—but possible. This vision is just that. It can only be possible if we all have a passion for relieving millions of people, present and future generations, from the pain and agony inflicted by the worst enemy we have ever faced.

The Vision of Victory

This book has given you the status of the war on cancer and the road to victory, at least from the perspectives of its author and contributors. You understand the magnitude of the problem. You know what has not happened and what needs to happen. You realize we are neither winning nor losing the war. We are at a stalemate, at a standoff, in a quagmire. Hopefully, you are beginning to see what you and millions of others must do, too. If the information in this book is taken to heart and enough people get intensely involved, we will see the cancer treatment pendulum begin to swing toward the direction of integrative medicine. When our population attains a healthy, balanced approach to cancer treatment, a definitive turn in the war will take place. When complementary treatments assume their proper role in the battle, victory will be in sight.

Everything that has been presented in this book has had the vision of a cancer free world as its backdrop. Most medical professionals, even some integrative medicine experts, don't believe cancer can ever be cured. They just want to make it as tolerable as possible and to increase its survivability rate. That is certainly a worthy goal. And, we will not even realize that goal without the help of universally practiced integrative medicine. Even if cancer proves to be an anomaly and cannot be cured, integrative treatment compared to conventional treatment is less toxic, less debilitating, less expensive, and less difficult to obtain and administer. However, I prefer to consider what happened to leprosy, smallpox, polio, and numerous other pandemic diseases throughout human history. In all of these cases, generations of people thought there would never be a cure. Let's expect nothing less than a cure.

The Political Vision

Since the political environment will have to change before much of anything else does, let's look at that part of the vision first. The future is a president's state of the union address which declares a substantial shift in strategy in the war on cancer. President Nixon declared the war. Now the vision sees a president who will end the quagmire and change the direction of the war. He lays out a multi-point plan for his Secretary of Health to pursue through the U.S. Department of Health and Human Services. He charges his Surgeon General to be a tireless spokesperson for the new strategy and to rally his commissioned corps to champion the movement. He schedules periodic news conference updates on the progress of the new cancer strategy. The president announces the following list as his top national health priority:

1.   A significant increase in the budget of the NCI

2.   One-third of the NCI budget for cancer research earmarked for CAM therapy research

3. Manpower and facilities of the NCI's Office of Cancer Complementary and Alternative Medicine (OCCAM) expanded 50%

4. Government grant incentives realigned to favor medical schools that make integrative medicine a substantial part of their required curriculum

5. Government grant incentives realigned to favor medical centers that conduct considerable CAM research

6. Lucrative tax incentives provided for pharmaceutical companies that create and develop new CAM products

7. Congress receives a presidential challenge to introduce legislation that levels the playing field for lobbying across the spectrum of the medical and pharmaceutical industries

8. A request from the president submitted for the AMA to modify its position on integrative medicine and to encourage its practice among AMA members

The Senate Majority Leader and the Speaker of the House lead their respective colleagues in pursuit of the following objectives:

1. Legislation that limits the activities, campaign contributions, and gifts of all lobbyists with particular attention to those from the medical and pharmaceutical industries

2. Passage of a bill that opens up competition significantly in the pharmaceutical market permitting the emergence of bona fide CAM entrepreneurs

3. An official proclamation urging the National Academy of Sciences to promote intense study of integrative cancer treatment

4. Pass the president's budget which increases the authorization for the NCI and earmarks a third for CAM therapy research

5. Expand patients' rights legislation to include options to demand and receive CAM therapies including evidence-based treatment not available in the U.S.

6. Passage of a bill that requires doctors to advise cancer patients of complementary therapy options and, to the extent qualified and willing, supply those treatments

7. Passage of a bill that requires health insurance companies to not discriminate between claims for evidence-based CAM therapies and conventional therapies

The Educational Vision

The 44 medical schools in the CAHCIM become the schools of choice for the majority of medical school applicants. These applicants learn through their premed courses that integrative medicine is the future direction of health care in America. Obtaining a degree from a prestigious medical school that strongly emphasizes integrative medicine provides a distinct advantage in competing for residence programs and ultimately in practice. The over 100 remaining medical schools that are not associated with CAHCIM see the trend and begin investing in the modification of their programs to include required studies in integrative medicine. Leading integrative medicine professors from CAHCIM schools become in high demand from the other schools. Medical educators across the country begin taking serious interest in integrative medicine.

Teaching medical centers emphasize integrative medicine in their residency programs. Specifically, new doctors choosing the oncology field begin their residency with wide-spread exposure to integrative oncology practice. New doctors are trained to allot sufficient time to each cancer patient while treating the patient rather than the disease. They learn the intricacies of nutrition, mind-body integration, spirituality, emotion, natural healing and other complements to conventional therapy. They practice under the tutelage of both integrative and conventional-only oncologists for a balanced perspective of cancer treatment.

Once residency is complete, all oncologists have ample opportunity to choose continuing education options that are deeply rooted in integrative oncology. Government agencies such as the NCI and IOM along with the SIO and other similar civil organizations provide numerous conferences and seminars for oncologists. All professionals in cancer treatment have far-reaching opportunities to hone their knowledge and skills in integrative concepts and techniques. The phrases integrative medicine and integrative health are used much less as all oncology practice assumes an integrative approach.

The Corporate Vision

Companies across the pharmaceutical industry realize the increasing public and governmental interest in exploring more integrative medicine options for cancer treatment. The companies see this as a needed shift in public relations and begin promotional support for such options. Modeled after the big oil companies' marketing campaign for alternative fuels and renewable energy, pharmaceutical ads emphasize their efforts toward developing non-toxic, natural products for cancer treatment. Instead of "going green" like the petroleum industry, the pharmaceutical industry seeks public sentiment by announcing that they are "going natural." As they continue to develop new chemically based drugs, the companies establish significant budget lines for research and clinical trials for natural, less harmful compounds. Even the stockholders of these companies realize the consumer goodwill gained from shifting some resources to the "natural" genre of cancer medicines. The expenses of this paradigm shift are offset by increased revenues from other products of the companies resulting from new marketing strategies. Companies add new departments completely dedicated to research and development of natural cancer treatment products.

Many medical centers and clinics tout their support for more natural solutions to complement all patient care, especially care of cancer patients. In many of their media ads, they promote themselves as having staff and policies that are natural medicine friendly. They highlight naturopathic doctors and integrative oncologists in their marketing efforts.

Retailers across the spectrum see the marketing advantage of demonstrating support for more natural solutions to cancer treatment. Many agree to sponsor fundraising efforts as a key complement to their marketing activities. Those that have a history of supporting cancer foundations and cancer centers support CAM treatment foundations and centers with effective CAM and integrative medicine programs. Marketing programs draw consumers by committing a portion of company profits to organizations active in the pursuit of integrative cancer research and treatment.

A logo is created which represents the integrative cancer research and development movement. This logo will eventually have the same degree of recognition as the pink ribbon. Its prominent display on products and advertisements acknowledges producers who are supporting the alternative movement financially. This logo will be a considerable incentive for consumers to purchase the product.

The Media Vision

To help the public capture the concept and buy in to the new strategy, both electronic and print media generate awareness and excitement as only they can. Lead stories about the new strategy are splashed on the covers of our most popular magazines, on the front page headlines of our major newspapers, and on home pages of news web sites. The raw facts about the debilitating and ubiquitous disease dominate articles by prominent columnists and feature writers. It becomes vogue to report on what will be the new paradigm in fighting the cancer war. The morning news shows like *Today, Fox and Friends, Good Morning America, American Morning*, and *The Early Show* as well as the evening network and cable news broadcasts produce short features on the new strategy. These shows routinely invite cancer experts to be interviewed often creating counterpoint debates between proponents of opposing views. Viewer surveys prove the insatiable interest in a new cancer strategy. Weekly programs such as *60 Minutes* and *Meet the Press* give viewers an inside look at new research and new policies of medical institutions that are legitimizing CAM therapies for cancer. News media reports will highlight particular corporations that support the integrative movement through their contributions and marketing programs. Reports emphasize companies that encourage customers to support integrative options through purchase of their products.

Hollywood and the music industry collectively take on the new strategy as one of their main social causes to advance. CAM research and freedom to choose treatments become the mantra that is repeated in awards ceremonies, movie debuts, and on music videos. With the intensity of Katie Couric's campaign against colon cancer, other celebrities specifically decry the present slowness of progress in the war and leverage their popularity to invoke action among their fans. A popular entertainment icon produces an annual telethon, ala Jerry Lewis, specifically for cancer research and treatment facilities with emphasis on CAM. Patterned after the 2008 star-studded *Stand Up to Cancer* telethon that appeared simultaneously on the big three networks, other telethons raise millions of dollars for research into CAM options. These highly publicized telethons will assure donors that much of the proceeds will fund the most promising integrative treatment efforts.

Individual Vision

Several individuals who have given millions of dollars to cancer research as well as education and treatment facilities have been named previously in this book. A few of these key philanthropists become convinced of the validity of more research at a higher level of sophistication for promising integrative treatment. Some agree to redistribute a percentage of their financial support to the field of integrative oncology. Others are compelled to completely shift their benevolence target to research of high potential CAM therapies. Still others who have not contributed previously to any cancer cause are convinced to begin major grants and endowments to the cause of integrative oncology.

At least one affluent business icon takes on a T. Boone Pickens-type role as a highly respected and visible advocate of greater dependence on opportunities outside traditional conventional cancer treatment. Mr. Pickens convinced millions of people of the critical need to lessen our dependence on foreign oil and to find alternative sources. Someone of like stature and credibility will convince millions of people of the critical need to lessen our exclusive dependence on conventional cancer treatment. He or she will reveal a plan to coordinate CAM research among pharmaceutical corporations, medical schools, and cancer centers.

Development of Past Visions

If this vision seems unreachable, it should. As I stated before, a worthwhile vision should be almost beyond comprehension, but possible. Seemingly impossible visions that were realized serve as inspirations. When the words, "I have a dream!" rang out from the steps of the Lincoln Memorial in 1963, a movement gained traction that changed the course of American culture. It wasn't just Martin Luther King, Jr. that propelled this nation-wide migration toward a higher virtue of civil rights. It was millions of people across the racial spectrum who became convicted and convinced of what was right. The vision was sparked by a few of relative insignificance, but taken up by many of powerful influence. We haven't arrived at the fullness of that vision yet. But, we have progressed further in it than anyone would have imagined in the unpredictable sixties.

At the risk of overusing another example, I must take us back to 1961 when America officially took up the gauntlet for the space race. A nation that had barely entered the jet age announced to the world its vision of putting a man on the moon in a decade. Impossible! Eight years later, the foot of an astronaut stamped the ingenuity of mankind into the dust of the moon's surface.

There are numerous other historical accounts of next-to-impossible visions that have been realized through the providence of God and the tenacity of man. All have two things in common, a belief that they could happen and a super-aggressive effort to make them happen. This is what it will take to realize the vision of the new strategy for the war on cancer.

CHAPTER 15

THE CALL FOR NEW WARRIORS

Remember from Chapter 1 that the cancer death toll is over 1500 per day. That equates to six fully-loaded 767 giant airliners crashing each day. In Chapter 2 we asked you to think about this statistic seriously as your read this book. Let's review the analogy now in a little more detail. If in one 24-hour period, terrorists brought down six huge airliners, what would happen? First, the FAA would ground all flying as it did on September 11, 2001. Secondly, the entire nation would turn its full attention and energies to the catastrophe.

What if, the next day, a major sports arena was hit on game day resulting in 1500 fatalities? Twenty-four hours later, another 1500 people were killed in a massive terrorist attack on another skyscraper office building. Then the day after, random shootings at shopping malls across the country took out 1500 more lives. As people stopped gathering anywhere in large groups, random shootings in cities, villages, and rural areas continued to lay claim to 1500 lives a day. Day after day, systematically, the best orchestrated, most sinister mass murder operation ever devised continued to sweep across our nation murdering 1500 each day. What would we do as a nation? How long would it take us to respond in a deliberate and effective way? A more poignant question: what would you do personally?

Terrorism is an elusive threat unlike any other threat to national sovereignty. It is not a defined national enemy that only attacks uniformed combatants. It indiscriminately attacks innocent civilians, and it blends undetectably into the population and cultural environment. Conventional warfare with massive troops, weapons of overwhelming destruction, and shock-and-awe tactics are ineffective against it. Unconventional warfare teams would have to be deployed throughout the country. Special operations tactics would have to be employed. Even then, it would be a tremendous task to stop such meticulously planned and implemented strikes across our homeland.

What if there was a call to arms for a militia-like army of private citizens to carry out specific assignments in combating the terrorists? If you were asked to drop everything, obtain a gun, use your vehicles, join a cell phone and internet communications network, and purchase whatever else was necessary for yourself and others, would you do it? Or, would you lock your doors, close the shades, and turn out the lights hoping you and your loved ones would somehow escape the reality of what was happening? Would you just depend on the powerful military establishment to protect you even though the 1500 deaths daily were continuing unabated? I want to believe that most of us would answer the call to arms.

This daily genocide-like scenario seems like the basis for a best-selling thriller novel or a box office smash hit. But, how is it different from what is actually happening in the real world in which we live? Instead of terrorism, it's cancer. Instead of our military that is ineffective against it, it's our conventional-only approach to treatment. Instead of our individual commitment to fight the terrorists unconventionally, it's the same level of individual commitment necessary to fight cancer unconventionally.

The human psyche is impossible to fully understand. We mere mortals will place our lives on the line to stop a society evil or catastrophe that shocks our very soul. Then, we just label as "an awful fact of life" something equally as horrendous and get on with our busy lives. The latter response is too often something that we have lived with so long that we have become hardened to it. It is no longer very offensive. The loss of 1500 lives a day to cancer is something most of us have lived with for all of our lives. It is in the background until it comes around to claim a parent, close relative, or dear friend. When it strikes close to home, we grieve with those we love, console them, and cry with them. When they are gone, we mourn for a while and put it behind us until death invades our circle again. The likelihood is that it will become very personal one day. The odds that any one of us will die of cancer is one in seven (Britt 2005). One in three of us will suffer with it, but a little over half of those inflicted will survive. Those odds are not good news, but perhaps worse is the fact that a cancer death is usually a premature death. It is also usually a long and agonizing way to die. Why do we accept these truths and respond by participating in an occasional race or periodically writing a small check to a cancer fund-raiser? If the deaths were caused by terrorists, we would be joining the military or on civil patrol packing heat.

It's Time to Enlist

For well over two centuries, our character and heritage as a nation has been to answer the call to arms when we have been attacked or threatened by a formidable enemy. Citizens always rallied in patriotic solidarity. Young men and women left their families, jobs, and schools to fight. Almost every able bodied man grabbed a musket and took the battle to the British in 1775. Over the next two centuries, millions of Americans were drafted to fight our domestic and international wars. Even the rather unpopular Iraq and Afghanistan wars with no draft saw thousands of brave souls respond to personal calls to duty for their country. Whether for independence, border protection, national security, or democracy abroad, almost everyone feels obligated to defend their loved ones and their way of life. Sadly, hundreds of thousands have had to pay the ultimate price. Table 15-1 gives us a somber account of those who gave their lives for their country (U. S. Department of Veteran Affairs 2009).

Table 15-1 Death Tolls of Major American Wars

War	Battle Deaths	Battle-related Deaths
American Revolution	4,435	17,000
War of 1812	2,260	?
Mexican American War	1,733	11,550
Civil War		
Union	140,414	224,097
Confederate	74,524[a]	59,297[a]
World War I	53,402	63,114
World War II	291,557	113,842
Korean War	33,741	2,833
Vietnam War	47,424	10,785
Iraq War	3,541[b]	834[b]
Afghanistan War	745[b]	233[b]
TOTAL	653,776	503,585
TOTAL BATTLE & BATTLE-RELATED	1,157,361	

a. Numbers based on insufficient records
b. Numbers at the time of this writing

Since its birth, our nation has lost over a million people in two centuries of major wars. That has been a heavy and regretful price to pay for our freedom and security. Over a million men and women left parents, children, other relatives, and close friends grieving and mourning their tragic losses. America lost over a million potential leaders and valuable contributors to our society.

Of course, I would not want to take anything from those who courageously sacrificed their lives for our life, liberty, and pursuit of happiness. As a career military veteran, I have the deepest respect and honor for those who purchased my freedom with their lives. But, let's consider another perspective. We have been fighting the war on cancer that is not listed in the table above. It has been going on for almost 40 years—about as long as the durations of all of our other major wars combined. Its casualty count is much higher than all of our other wars combined—much, much higher. In fact, about as many die in the cancer war every two years as have died in our nation's entire history of wars. Over 18 million people have fallen on the cancer war battlegrounds since the war began in 1971 (National Center for Health Statistics [NCHS] 2008). That is 16 times more cancer deaths during the four-decade war on cancer than the number of deaths from all of our nation's major military wars combined.

In Chapter 1, Table 1-1 revealed how little the mortality rate for cancer had changed over the duration of the war. Now, let's look at how little the actual number of cancer deaths have changed at five-year points during the same period (Table 15-2) (National Center for Health Statistics (NCHS 2008). Keep in mind the relativity of these numbers based on population growth.

Table 15-2   U. S. Cancer Deaths Annually

Year	Deaths
1971	336,005
1975	364,111
1980	416,509
1985	461,563
1990	505,322
1995	538,455
2000	553,888
2005	559,312

So, where is the outrage? Where is the public outcry that this war has to end, and end in victory? Where are the volunteer recruits ready to take up arms and win the war? It begins with you. This is an appeal for you to do whatever it takes to help defeat perhaps the greatest enemy our society has ever faced. It is a call for you, armed with fresh knowledge and resolute determination, to become an activist in fighting cancer. You will not be dodging bullets and bombs, but you will probably meet opposition from some of the cancer treatment traditionalists. You will not be a full-time soldier, but you will have to re-prioritize your time.

You will not win medals, but you will receive a lot of personal fulfillment. You will not be assigned a certain unit and combat skill, but you will need to choose your battle ground based on your personal skills and passions.

There are almost unlimited opportunities for action in this war. Some of you may only be able to participate in one area. In that case, I urge you to immerse yourself in that area and become an expert and possibly a leader. Others may have the ability to serve in several different areas. In those cases, order your activities wisely placing priorities according to relative needs and critical timing. Still others may not be able to participate in any activities, but can support the activities financially. In those cases, please give liberally to organizations and projects that support the integrative treatment strategy such as those listed in Appendix B.

Every movement in humankind that has had a lasting positive impact on society has begun with a handful of people devoted to a common cause. Two millennia ago, twelve ragtag disciples organized a movement that changed the world for eternity. Far less significant, but nonetheless noteworthy, was a "committee of five" whose 1863 collaboration in Geneva, Switzerland, led to today's International Committee of the Red Cross with societies in nearly every country of the world. Nancy Brinker promised her sister who was dying of cancer that she would do everything possible to find a cure for the disease. With the help of a few friends and relatives, she founded the Susan G. Komen Foundation—a name recognized by almost every American today. Margaret Mead said, "Never doubt that a small group of thoughtful, committed citizens can change the world; indeed it's the only thing that ever has."

Five Responses to the Cancer Crisis

Everyone is living out their response to the global crisis of cancer in some way. There can be no such thing as not responding to any crisis. Not taking any kind of action is itself a response. Everyone who knows about the horrors of cancer, and that's every sane adult, chooses one of the following personal responses:

Intimidation: It's too big for me to do anything about.

Cancer is a formidable enemy. However, common people taking on uncommon tasks have defeated giants throughout the centuries. Moses, David, Joan of Arc, and Abraham Lincoln are eclectic examples of individuals from humble beginnings who have literally changed history. The discovery of new continents, the defeat of despot monarchies, the industrial revolution, and the conquering of space represent "impossibilities" made possible by mere people who could not accept the status quo.

Isolation: If I ignore it, it will go away.

It is easy to just not acknowledge a problem that seems unmanageable. This happened in the holocaust, and it didn't go away. It happened with America before entering World War II, and we were almost too late. It allowed terrorism to go unchecked during the years leading up to 9-11, and we are still suffering the consequences. It permitted financial and industrial institutions worldwide to implode in 2008 and 2009, and the aftershock will be passed to future generations. Denial doesn't solve anything, it just postpones the solution. Denial by one person almost always produces prolonged pain for another. The same is true of one generation's effect on another generation.

Substitution: Someone else can do it better than I.

The first sarcastic question in human history was, "Am I my brother's keeper?" Since then, a common rejection to calls for help has been to shirk personal responsibility and to pass it along to someone else. Something could always seemingly be done better by someone else with more skill, time, resources, and energy. Truth is, the people most successful at bringing about life-changing improvements are those who have the most passion for the change regardless of perceived ability.

Resignation: I just have to live with it; nothing is going to change.

In every circumstance of life, we choose how to react: as the victim of the outcome or the determiner of the outcome. Unfortunately, there are more defeatists in the world than activists. Helen Keller said, "Science may have found a cure for most evils; but it has found no remedy for the worst of them all—the apathy of human beings." Apathy about cancer is worse than cancer itself. Some people will always survive cancer, but no one will avoid the potential of cancer as long as apathy toward its eradication prevails.

Confrontation: I must do something.

The only positive response to the crisis of cancer is confrontation. We cannot just leave it to the physicians and medical scientists to confront the disease. This formidable enemy will only be defeated if millions of us enlist in the war effort. Confrontation comes in the form of greater awareness, pursuit of broader therapy options, patient participation in treatment decisions, financial support for new research projects, challenges to the pharmaceutical industry and education institutions, and political activism. Put simply, we must confront the status quo. We must reject all convenient responses to cancer and choose confrontation.

Where Do You Stand?

It is not the purpose of this chapter to put you on a guilt trip. No cause should ever be taken on from a feeling of guilt. No one should be drawn into this new strategy movement based on external pressure. Whatever you set your mind to should come from a well informed, well thought through process of decision making. It should come from a sense of passion and an unquenchable drive to help change something monumental. If the motivation does not come from within, it should be dismissed. This entire book has attempted to provide the unabridged information necessary for independent thinking and decision making to implement a new strategy for the war on cancer. Equipping readers for waging this war has been my objective. It's now up to you.

Albert Schweitzer said, "Civilization can only revive when there shall come into being in a number of individuals a new tone of mind, independent of the prevalent one among the crowds, and in opposition to it—a tone of mind which will gradually win influence over the collective one, and in the end determine its character."

So, what will <u>you</u> do, specifically? Please allow me to encourage you to become active in three objectives.

First, if you agree with the new strategy, you should want to take steps to <u>solidify your personal commitment</u> to its objectives in your own health and medical decisions.

Then, if you believe the new strategy is in the best interests of everyone touched by cancer, you should help <u>generate action within political, educational, corporate, and media institutions; and among individuals</u>.

Finally, if you realize that the strategy's success depends on sufficient resources, you should be willing to help <u>raise the funds necessary</u>.

Venues for these objectives are the subject matter for the next chapter.

CHAPTER 16

THE VENUES FOR BATTLE

There are areas of your life and places in your environment that serve as the most productive battlegrounds for your fight. Every campaign begins with a plan. I encourage you to take the time to plan which part of your life you can redirect toward the new strategy. Decide where your talents and skills can be most effectively used. Then refer to this chapter as a guide to effectively carry out the plan.

Commit Personally

The key to success in accomplishing anything worthwhile is commitment. If a new strategy for the war on cancer is to become reality, thousands of people across this land must make it their personal battle. Your personal commitment to the vision cast in this book will combine with others with like passion to raise up a formidable force. Here is what you can do specifically.

Educate Yourself

Preparing yourself for battle in this war requires your being very knowledgeable and well equipped. Hopefully, this book gives you a fundamental foundation on which to build your personal education in the new strategy. But, you will need a lot more understanding of integrative cancer treatment, its advantages, and its challenges. I recommend you develop a structured reading program involving books, articles, and news items involving integrative medicine in general and integrative cancer treatment in specific. Search your local library and the internet for recent books that are available on the subject. Take considerable time to surf the internet, letting search engines take you to an almost endless number of Web sites dealing with CAM and integrative medicine. Be alert for breaking news in all media that will give you the latest information on subjects related to the new strategy. You can, in a fairly short time, become an expert in many aspects of integrative medicine. Knowledge is power when it comes to communicating with your medical providers about your health or the health of your loved ones.

Take Responsibility

Take personal responsibility for understanding, and sometimes directing, the medical care you are getting. Be very transparent with your doctor about any CAM practices you are engaged in. If you are given any prescription medication, discuss with your doctor any and all supplements you are taking or unconventional health practices you are doing. Make sure there are no incompatibilities with what your doctor prescribes. If there is any question about any indicator of potential cancer, get a second opinion from another doctor. Don't wait a prolonged period for your doctor to order a second X-ray or blood test for comparison with a previous one. Request a shorter period for comparison or see another doctor. If you are diagnosed with cancer, tell your doctor that you insist on treatment by integrative practitioners. During treatment by an integrative oncologist, ensure that you maintain a constant dialogue about your treatment and understand your options fully.

Get Involved

Step beyond your commitment to yourself into a commitment to your family, friends, and everyone who will face the darkness of cancer. Make the personal decision to confront this disease rather than be intimidated by it, isolated from it, or resigned to it. One person cannot do everything, but everyone can do something.

Generate Action

Just becoming knowledgeable will not have an impact beyond your own circle. It is essential that you become a catalyst for generating action among others, especially others with influence.

Challenge Politicians

Contact Government Officials

The president is the ultimate policy maker in this country. During the presidential campaigns, the public can begin to influence future cancer policy by making it a campaign issue. Integrative cancer treatment advocates should attend campaign forums and ask questions that hold the candidate accountable for a new strategy. Once a president is elected, you can influence the cabinet appointments, particularly the Health and Human Services Secretary, through your senators who approve them. Well into the administration's term of office, letters and petitions to the president have an impact.

Not only do our United States congressmen and senators pass the budget for the NIH and NCI, the largest source for cancer research funding, but they also control wide-ranging health care policy. Little of significance will happen toward the new strategy until the Congress takes specific actions in that direction. Your first step is becoming more politically active in this effort is to obtain the contact information for your two senators and your congressman. Send them emails, call their Washington offices as well as their local offices, and write them letters. Send them articles, Web site address, even books that will inform them of the integrative oncology movement. Yes, send them each a new copy of this book! Enlist the help of your friends and relatives in this effort. Politicians do read and respond to communications from their constituents. Don't stop after one series of contacts. Set up a periodic plan for making subsequent contacts. Perhaps one contact each month through rotating mediums of communication would be appropriate. Be persistent, but don't be a pest.

Chapter 14 included the political vision for the new strategy. Review it and develop your own personal strategy for your part in fulfilling that vision. Ask your legislators, federal and state, to support the elements of the vision. For instance, request that they initiate or support an increase in the budget for the NCI with one-third of the budget targeted at complementary therapy research. Ask them to expand the NCI's OCCAM by 50%. Seek limitations on lobbying and gifts by the pharmaceutical companies and medical agencies. Encourage policies that provide patient access to and insurance payment for integrative cancer treatments.

Maintain contact with the members of the Senate Committee on Health, Education, Labor, and Pensions. This is the legislative hub for medical bills and budgets. In the Executive Branch, the U. S. Department of Health and Human Services should be contacted and urged to make integrative medicine a prime public information priority.

Work in Campaigns

We often hear that we should not vote for political candidates based on their position on a single issue. That is probably wise counsel in general. However, if a candidate's position on an issue violates the very core of our values, that position alone should be grounds for casting the ballot for another contender. If a candidate opposes, or at least does not support, something that we feel is vital to our way of life, we should not only vote for, but campaign for, another candidate who supports it. If it is an issue that is extremely important to us, we have a duty to help the candidate who favors our position in every way we can.

If the new cancer strategy advocated by this book is truly important to you, you should be adamant about determining which politician will actively support it and which will not. Our first concern should be presidential candidates. We need a president who will vow to achieve victory in the war on cancer. Part of his or her platform should be to appoint cabinet secretaries in departments of Health and Human Services and the Treasury who will aggressively pursue the new strategy with necessary policy and funding. The potential president should promise to appoint a Surgeon General who has a heart for integrative medicine. The strategy should have a prominent place in his campaign rhetoric. His campaign health care advisors should embrace integrative medicine. A presidential hopeful who makes this an important part of his or her campaign is worthy of more than our vote. He or she is worthy of our campaign involvement and monetary contributions.

Actively campaigning for congressional candidates with these attributes is also very important. We should ask the question directly of any prospective representative or senator, "Will you heartily pursue the advancement of integrative medicine?" At least make them take a position and not get a pass on the subject. If a candidate agrees with you, actively campaign for him or her. Then, if he or she wins, be a constant reminder of the commitment.

Don't underestimate the importance of state-level politics. States have a lot to say about what is and is not allowed in the way of health care. States are almost autonomous in their budgets for Medicaid and its levels of coverage. Governors and state legislators, even attorneys general, need to feel the pressure to support the new strategy. If any of these candidates in your state show a willingness to further the causes of integrative medicine, especially as it applies to cancer therapy, volunteer to help get them elected.

Challenge Medical Educators

As discussed in previous chapters, a few medical schools are making progress as advocates of integrative medicine. Universities that form the CAHCIM are to be commended for their lead in this area. However, as we saw in Chapter 12, the great majority of medical schools in America have little or no curricula that allow medical students to develop the slightest understanding of an integrative approach to health care. The new strategy for the war on cancer cannot become reality until our nation experiences a fundamental change in how we educate our physicians, more specifically our oncologists.

The Bravewell Collaborative, a philanthropic organization for advancing public health and wellness, describes this fundamental change in the core curriculum used to train medical students as the most critical need identified by physician leaders. Some of the barriers to education that they identify are segmentation of medicine into specialties, overemphasis on technology and pharmaceuticals, and ignorance of prevention strategies and integrative modalities that add value to health care (Bravewell Collaborative 2009). It is clear to Bravewell philanthropists that changing medical education and training is essential to sustain movement toward integrative medicine. They are already supporting infrastructure and curriculum development for CAHCIM schools. Willing donors are ready to fund more of the integrative medicine movement. Public support for the movement in institutes of higher learning is now a critical aspect of this funding.

Now is the time for you to make contact with the medical schools in your area and any others with which you have association. The most appropriate contact would be the dean of academics. Ask them to become more familiar with the CAHCIM and its member schools. Have the CAHCIM Web address, www. imconsortium.org, available to offer. Recommend the CAHCIM paper outlining curriculum recommendations for their schools which can be downloaded from the Bravewell Collaborative Web site, www.bravewell.org. Suggest that the dean assign a department staff member to provide a report on what is happening in integrative medicine, particularly in the medical schools arena. Encourage the dean to take a personal interest in integrative medicine and to become the catalyst for its inclusion in the school's core curriculum. Ask him or her how you can personally help with this change. Of course, as always, do your homework in familiarizing yourself with these resources before contacting the medical school.

Challenge Corporations

How to become involved in this category is probably the least obvious of the bunch. But, it's not that hard. You don't really have to be an Erin Brockovich to be effective in helping change corporate behavior. Companies are sensitive to public opinion and customer desires. That's why they all have public relations departments and customer service departments. They change as the culture and the market change. A fundamental principle in a capitalist economy is that households, the basic unit of the free market, determine what is produced. Remember a few years ago when the oil companies just wanted to sell more gasoline. That's all their advertising was about. More recently, as the public interest switched toward alternative fuels, the Exxon Mobils, Royal Dutch Shells, and BPs of the world are almost exclusively touting their advances in alternative fuels. That has to happen in pharmaceuticals, medical institutions, and health insurance.

Pharmaceutical Companies

We know what is driving a corporation by how it advertises. Over the last few years, the major pharmaceutical corporations have been spending a lot of advertising dollars to convince us to demand their brand of products from our providers. The television entices us to "ask your doctor if (fill in the blank) is right for you." Internet pop-ups flash with the latest prescription drug available for whatever ails us. Newspapers and magazines print full-page ads touting new prescription drugs along with an accompanying section of fine print with all the scientific details and side effects. Why is this important to the pharmaceutical companies? Because they realize that it is the general public that they are going to have to convince, not the doctors and other health professionals. It is the person who is sick and asks their doctor for a specific drug that is going to make their sales. Sure the good looking sales reps who make pitches and leave samples for the doctors play a big role in drug promotion and sales. But, the drug makers know that, if the patient asks for it, the doctors are likely to prescribe it.

So, what needs to happen is for patients to begin asking for complementary, non-pharmaceutical medicines and other treatments. If enough newly diagnosed cancer patients asked for natural treatments to complement their conventional therapies, oncologists would begin getting the message. When an oncologist starts explaining the chemotherapy, radiation, or surgery protocol that he or she was about to prescribe, the patient should ask what diet, supplemental vitamins, pain-reducing acupuncture, meditation, exercise, detoxification, immune system enhancement, etc. that he or she would be recommending along with it. Ask what natural, non-chemical enhancements he would suggest to boost the conventional therapy and reduce its side effects. In time, that would encourage doctors to get smarter in those integrative practices and would motivate pharmaceutical companies to get more serious about research and development in those areas.

Can you envision a full-page ad by a major pharmaceutical company that showcases its recent breakthrough in developing a grape seed extract product that appears to render cancer cells completely vulnerable to chemotherapy? The ad might proudly promise that cancer sufferers and caregivers could count on their company to develop natural, non-toxic medicines and methods to fight cancer. If grassroots America became vocal enough in their impatience with lack of choice in treatment options, the pharmaceutical industry would respond with more options. It would become a public relations necessity.

Too long our excuse has been that the industry will never seriously research natural options because there is no return on investment. They won't spend money exploring the potential benefits of that grape seed extract, we lament, because, if it works, how can they make billions from such a plentiful product? Two things are wrong with that assumption. First, although clinical trials of a common natural substance would be less costly, the trial sponsor would have less invested be recouped, therefore, creating an opportunity for less risks and greater profits. Secondly, a company that discovers and develops such a natural treatment breakthrough deserves its patent right. Once a patent is obtained, the company has a virtual monopoly and is only bound in its pricing by government regulation and professional restraints. Granted, once the industry began to collectively see the economic sense of natural product research, competition would drive prices lower because of cheaper raw ingredients. But companies would be on a level playing field, and profit margins would be maintained.

So, the only way to change the focus of pharmaceutical companies is for patients and caregivers to demand natural-based complementary options for treatment. That starts at the first visit to any oncologist who is not willing or capable of offering integrative treatment.

Medical Centers and Clinics

Every advocate of this new strategy should pursue the establishment of one or more integrative oncologists in each cancer treatment center or clinic in his or her local area. If you have a circle of friends who are passionate about the need for a new strategy for the war on cancer, meet with them to plan this pursuit. If you don't have such a group, organize one. You need the support of others to be effective in any kind of advocacy activity. One person may be perceived as a wacko. A small group is seen as a fledgling movement. Conduct a telephone or email survey of all cancer centers, cancer clinics, hospital cancer departments, or oncologist groups. Find out which have few or no integrative therapy options. Carry out a well organized campaign to influence the inclusion of integrative therapy options in those organizations that lack the capability. Determine which one or two seem the most receptive and focus all efforts in that direction. Recommend that the organization add an integrative oncologist position. If necessary, circulate petitions throughout the community and present the organizations with many pages of signatures representing those who desire integrative options to be introduced into their local area. Be creative. Use the news media. Write letters to the editor of newspapers. Meet with your local chamber of commerce officials and urge them to recruit an integrative oncology clinic for your city. If nothing else, that will motivate the existing clinics and centers to consider hiring an integrative oncologist in order to discourage competition.

If an integrative oncologist or oncology center establishes itself in your community, become the new service's best advocate. Host a welcome party and invite prominent guests who will hear what the new concept in cancer treatment is all about. Explore opportunities for promoting the service through various media. Enlist a group of volunteers to assist the new doctor or doctors. If the new service is ushered in by a positive manner in which the community is unaccustomed, it will benefit greatly by the special attention.

Grocery and Food Services

As integrative oncology options are developed in your community, concurrent emphases must be placed on healthy food availability. Cancer patients will be placed on nutrition plans that necessitate an abundance of fresh, organic vegetables and fruits. For too many communities, such commodities, if available at all, are only found at high prices in specialty stores. Major supermarkets must be lobbied to carry more cancer-patient-friendly products free of potential carcinogens and high in vitamin and mineral content. Such foods are important for cancer prevention, but critical for cancer therapy.

Likewise, restaurants, especially fast food restaurants, should be urged to offer fresh, organic selections on their menus. Patients undergoing cancer therapy will often be unable to cook or even be around the kitchen. Forced to eat out often, these consumers deserve to have a full range of food possibilities that will fit their therapy plan. Concentrate on at least one nice restaurant and one fast food location that can be convinced to custom-make a few cancer-patient-friendly menu items and promote them as such.

Challenge the Media

Television, Newspaper, and Internet

Whether electronic or print, the news media are always looking for interesting stories. Make it your goal to feed them unique and current news items related to integrative cancer therapies. Become a reliable source and an expert in what is happening on the new ideas front for cancer. If your local news hasn't featured this book yet, take them a copy and explain its content as newsworthy. Point them to other publications promoting integrative treatment. Seek out a cancer survivor who has benefited from integrative options, preferably local, and encourage the news media to interview him or her. Help set up a news interview with the nearest integrative oncologist. If the oncologist is a distance from the local community, make that an issue in the story.

Often, newspapers welcome submitted articles. If you have a talent for writing, write your own article highlighting the new strategy for the war on cancer and turn it in with a cover letter requesting its publication. Write an *Op-Ed* piece registering your frustration with the insufficiency of integrative medicine capability within your community. At least write a simple letter to the editor for publication which often gets a point-counterpoint going for days. After reading this book, you should find it easy to enter into debate on the editorial page of your newspaper.

Hollywood

The stars of the film industry in America occasionally become spokespersons for the cancer war. It is fashionable for celebrities, and it resonates with their fans. Also, when a cinema elite is diagnosed with the disease, it explodes on the front pages of magazines and tabloids. So, famous actors coming from various angles are routinely high visibility symbols for the cure.

Unfortunately for integrative oncology, most cancer activists from the Hollywood scene advocate exclusively for the ACS, Komen, or a particular center. Their efforts are almost entirely directed toward finding a better drug or funding a facility. Even the few stars who have benefited from integrative or alternative therapy are not prone to become a high profile advocate for it. About the only celebrity who has been a public ambassador for integrative cancer treatment is Suzanne Somers, a cancer survivor who credits natural hormone therapy for her continuing remission. Celebrity is a hard domain for a common person to enter, but its impact would always be worth every effort. I suggest getting involved in fan clubs or fan social networks through which you could influence fans and others close to particular celebrities. Anything that would pique the interest of the rich and famous in the new strategy would be an advantage. The natural and non-toxic aspects of integrative therapy should be well received in the environmentally sensitive culture of Hollywood. If you have a little "groupie" fascination with the celebrity life, you might make some significant inroads into that world. If Hollywood took up the cause of integrative cancer treatment, it would be a huge breakthrough.

Challenge Individuals

Philanthropy

Hard reality is that anything worthwhile comes at a great cost. It costs time and effort, but additionally it always costs money. If the worthwhile endeavor is outside the mainstream of public thinking or has organized opposition, its cost is far greater. The cost of implementing the new strategy in time and effort of individuals as described in this chapter is substantial. But, the funding of research and public information projects is equally substantial. Fundraising activities, thousands of individual donations, along with public and private grants are essential to the new strategy's success. However, like any other major movement, some very significant financial support from affluent philanthropists is absolutely necessary for victory in the cancer war. Specific research projects must capture the hearts of particular philanthropists who will become passionate about the works and underwrite them from start to finish.

This is another area where new strategy supporters can be of tremendous assistance. Almost everyone knows personally, is acquainted with, or otherwise has access to someone whose sizable financial gifts fund favorite charitable causes. If you can make any kind of connection with persons who graciously share their wealth for the good of others, I encourage you to do so. Usually, they just need to be apprised of the need and how their gifts will be used. Your passion for the cause will be infectious. The prospect of helping win a war that is killing over 1500 innocent people a day and causing many thousands more to suffer is convincing in itself. Act as a representative of one of the non-profit organizations listed in the appendix of this book that supports research and development of integrative cancer therapy. Become familiar with the organization, so you can present its objectives in a professional manner. Provide information and materials to the philanthropist and follow through with whatever process he or she requires. Your introduction of the new strategy to someone who could fund an entire research project could ultimately save many lives and improve the quality of life for thousands of cancer sufferers. This is an opportunity to vastly multiply what you might be able to accomplish for the new strategy on your own.

Business Leaders

A distinct advantage in the advancement of integrative cancer care would be public support from a few business leaders of national prominence. Men and women who have a solid reputation for business sense would catch the attention of both the general public and the medical community. It would also discredit the assumption that, if a therapy did not provide a monetary return on investment for business, it cannot make it to the clinical trials. These icons of industry would be espousing that not everything has to produce income. Some investment returns come in the form of altruism. They could also testify that victory over cancer is well worth any sacrifice from the business world. This message would particularly ring clear for those in the pharmaceutical industry. As mentioned in Chapter 14, the advocacy of oil magnate T. Boone Pickens for alternative energy sources is a model for a renowned business leader's advocacy of the new strategy. What if the CEO of one of the largest drug companies made frequent appearances throughout the media proposing a plan to establish hundreds of new integrative oncology centers across the nation and many new research labs exclusively for integrative medicine?

Some of you work in a national or international corporation whose CEO or president is recognized nationally. You may or may not have any kind of access to the front office of the headquarters. But, you could at least get the attention of your company's top officials with letters that have more influence than others because you work for the company. Send the CEO or president materials and web site addresses that will stir their interest in the subject. At an appropriate point, ask one of them to become a spokesperson for integrative oncology. You could be the catalyst that produces a T. Boone Pickens for integrative oncology.

Raise Funds

Underwriting a strategy of this magnitude might seem almost impossible. The only way it is possible is through the dedicated efforts of many to multiply their own capabilities in many others. By providing opportunities for others to contribute their resources, your potential for raising funds exponentially is almost unlimited.

Designate Funds for Integrative Therapy

Self-initiated Fundraising

There are more ways to raise funds for a charitable cause than we can possible cover in this chapter. Fun runs, fun walks, bike trips, yard sales, bake sales, auctions, door to door canvassing, and mass mailings are just a few types of projects that are consistently successful. The important stipulation is that the funds contributed will be used exclusively in the advancement of integrative cancer treatment.

You know your comfort levels and abilities for raising charitable funds. Of course, you may need to get outside of your comfort zone, but you will need to operate within your own abilities. Evaluate your circle of friends and your community to determine what is popular and has proven successful in past fundraising activities. Then recruit a group to help you organize the best activity and go for it.

Recipients for the funds raised can be local, regional, or national. Perhaps a local cancer clinic or medical educational facility can use the funds for integrative oncology related projects or equipment. You may have an integrative oncology center in your state or region that has a capital development need. The not-for-profit foundations in the appendix of this book that exclusively support integrative oncology research and projects are certainly appropriate choices for funds raised or personal contributions.

Structured Fundraising Projects

Most foundations and some other organizations that support integrative oncology have structured fundraising project plans. These plans make it much easier to initiate and conduct a project. For instance, one of the core fundraising opportunities for my Connie Thompson Foundation is the "New Again" community yard sale. Plans and materials for the project are pre-packaged and available for any person or group that wants to conduct a convenient and successful fundraiser for integrative oncology. Other organizations have similar packages.

Stick to Your Niche

After you have served in a particular venue, evaluate your success and satisfaction with it. If it doesn't fulfill your passion or meet your expectations, you may want to transition to another area. It is important that you find the venue that you enjoy and brings positive results. Once that has been determined, enrich your talents and skills there and stick with it.

If you continue to change venues often, you will not likely gain the expertise and experience that you need to be most effective and efficient in any venue. To realize the greatest potential for advancing the cause, you will need to develop your abilities and influences as the "go to" person in your singular area of service. For instance, if you are best at generating action in the political arena, strive to become the best political activist you can be. If you are better at fundraising, try to set the standard for that effort.

I urge you to enlist in the war, to choose your battle ground, to hone your abilities for the fight, and to accept nothing short of victory. It will be worth the price.

AFTERWORD

As you finish this book, my hope and prayer is that it has made a difference in your thinking and priorities. Armed with more knowledge and greater passion for defeating cancer, you now have the opportunity to be a part of the new strategy essential to victory. This new strategy will at least prolong life, increase quality of life, and significantly reduce treatment side effects for cancer victims. It could at most defeat cancer as we know it.

Many types of complementary cancer therapies have been proven to produce a relatively normal quality of life during conventional treatment. With therapies that ensure fewer debilitating side effects, patients can more easily manage their healing. With physical, psychological, and spiritual enhancements, they can more aggressively devote their body, mind, and soul to healing. These advantages have been known to help extend the lives of cancer patients, often to a typical life span. If these results alone were universally realized, all of the efforts to implement the new strategy would be more than justified.

The higher vision of this strategy, however, is to ultimately defeat this monstrous enemy. As the strategy is implemented on a grand scale, we will have more researchers in more laboratories experimenting with more natural, non-toxic options. We will have more oncologists finding success with more therapies that do no harm. We will have more cancer patients insisting on complementary therapies. All of this will generate burgeoning scientific data bases to support a wave of clinical trials for complementary and alternative therapies. Once the new paradigm of research and treatment is established, new concepts and formulas will be widely debated and tested. I believe this will ultimately produce the breakthrough that we have been seeking for decades. It may be a something that naturally kills tumors, prevents cell mutations, alters chromosomes, fosters immunity, or heals in a way we've never imagined.

The new strategy for the war on cancer brings victory either way. It could very possibly lead to an end to the disease. Failing that, it will make the disease much more tolerable than ever before. It is clear that a new strategy is essential. If the answer to cancer were only in further drug research and the exclusive practice of conventional treatment, cancer would be relegated to the history books by now.

So, who will initiate this new strategy? We will. All of us who are convinced it is the only hope for defeating cancer will implement it from wherever we are. Most national strategies begin from the government, industry, or academia. All three shape our culture and will play a role in implementing this strategy. However, if it were going to originate from those sources, it would have already done so. This has to be a grass roots strategy comparable to the civil rights movement.

The cost of delay is too high at over 1500 lives per day in America. We can't accept 40 more years of the status quo in this war. We should refuse to accept one more year. Without abandoning the good of conventional treatment, we must reach for the best of integrative treatment. Let's do it! Now!

ABOUT THE AUTHOR

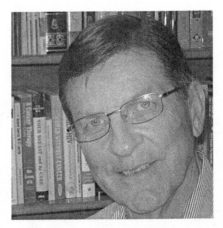

Terry Thompson graduated from the University of Arkansas and received his MBA from the University of Oklahoma City. After retiring as a colonel in the U.S. Air Force, he served nine years as a staff pastor in a large church. He later became the general manager of a nationally syndicated outdoor sports television program. A professor for John Brown University, he teaches in the Business Division Advance Program. He recently published a book, *The Aviator's Devotional*, which has been very popular among aviation enthusiasts. In 2001, Terry lost his wife of 33 years to cancer after three years of agonizing battle with the disease. He has established a cancer research foundation in her name, The Connie Thompson Foundation. The dark-valley experience of living with cancer drove him to research the state of America's cancer treatment and pursue a new treatment strategy. Terry manages two web sites, www.newcancerstrategy.com for this book and www.cancerchoices. org for the Foundation. He keeps blogs current on both sites with intriguing and provoking insights. Terry and his wife, Linda, have four children and six grandchildren between them. They reside in Hot Springs, Arkansas.

APPENDIX A

The following list of integrative oncology centers and clinics is not exhaustive, but rather a reference of providers of complementary cancer treatments readily available at the time of publication. Criteria for the listing include a certified integrative oncologist at the facility. The author assumes no responsibility for the accuracy or credibility of the organizations. Updates to this list may be obtained at and submitted to <u>www.cancerchoices.org</u>.

Block Center for Integrative
Cancer Care
1800 Sherman Ave.
Evanston, IL 60201
847-492-3040
<u>www.blockmd.com</u>

Buchholz Medical Group
1174 Castro St., Suite 275
Mountain View, CA 94040
<u>www.buchholzmedgroup.com</u>
650-988-8011

Cancer Treatment Centers of America
14200 W. Fillmore St.
Goodyear, AZ 85338
<u>www.cancercenter.com/western-hospital.cfm</u>
800-268-0786

Cancer Treatment Centers of America
1331 E. Wyoming Ave.
Philadelphia, PA 19124
<u>www.cancercenter.com/eastern-hospital.cfm</u>
800-268-0786

Cancer Treatment Centers of America
900 SW 16th St.
Renton, WA 98057
www.cancercenter.com/seattle-clinic.cfm
800-268-0786

Cancer Treatment Centers of America
10109 E. 79th St.
Tulsa, OK 74113
www.cancercenter.com/southwestern-hospital.cfm
800-268-0786

Cancer Treatment Centers of America
2520 Elisha Ave.
Zion, IL 60099
www.cancercenter.com/midwestern-hospital.cfm
800-268-0786

The Center for Integrative Medicine at University of Colorado
1635 Aurora Court, 5th Floor
Aurora, CO 80045
www.uch.edu
720-848-0000

The Center for Integrative Medicine at George Washington University
908 New Hampshire Ave., Ste. 200
Washington, DC 20037
www.integrativemedicinedc.com
202-833-5055

Center for Women's Health
Oregon Health and Science University
3181 S. W. Sam Jackson Park Rd.
Portland, OR 97239
www.ohsu.edu/cam
503-418-4500

Century Wellness Clinic
521 Hammill Ln.
Reno, NV 89511
www.drforsythe.com
775-827-0707

Duke Integrative Medicine
3475 Erwin Rd.
Durham, NC 27705
www.dukeintegrativemedicine.org
919-660-6826

Gaynor Integrative Oncology
215 East 72nd St.
New York, NY 10021
www.gaynoroncology.com
212-472-2828

Goshen Center for Cancer Care
200 High Park Ave.
Goshen, IN 46526
www.goshenhealth.org
866-496-4673

Johns Hopkins CAM Center
1813 E. Monument St.
Baltimore, MD 21287
www.hopkinsmedicine.org
410-614-5678

M. D. Anderson Integrative
Medicine Program
1515 Holcombe Blvd. Unit 16
Houston, TX 77030
www.mdanderson.org
713-794-4700

Memorial Sloan-Kettering Cancer
Center, Integrative Medicine
1275 York Ave.
New York, NY 10065
www.mskcc.org
212-639-2000

Naturemed Integrative Medicine
5330 Manhattan Circle, Suite B
Boulder, CO 80303
www.naturemedclinic.com
303-884-7557

Osher Clinical Center for
Complementary and Integrative
Medical Therapies
Brigham and Women's Hospital
850 Boylston St.
Chestnut Hill, MA 02467
www.brighamandwomens.org/
medicine/oshercenter
617-732-9700

Rocky Mountain Cancer Centers
7951 E. Maplewood Ave., Ste. 300
Greenwood Village, CO 80111
www.rockymountaincancercenters.
com
888-259-7622

Simms/Mann UCLA Center for
Integrative Oncology
200 UCLA Medical Plaza, Suite 502
Los Angeles, CA 90095
www.simmsmanncenter.ucla.edu
310-794-6644

Stanford Center for Integrative
Medicine
1101 Welch Rd, Ste. A6
Stanford, CA 94305
www.stanfordhospital.org
650-498-5566

UCLA Center for Integrative
Oncology
200 UCLA Medical Plaza, Ste. 502
Los Angeles, CA 90095
www.ccim.med.ucla.edu
310-794-6644

UCSF Osher Center for Integrative
Medicine
1701 Divisadero St., Ste 150
San Francisco, CA 94115
www.osher.ucsf.edu
415-353-7720

UM Sylvester Comprehensive
Cancer Center
1475 NW 12th Ave.
Miami, FL 33136
www.sylvester.org
305-243-1000

Valley Cancer Institute
12099 W. Washington Blvd., Ste. 304
Los Angeles, CA 90066
www.vci.org
310-398-0013

Western Washington Oncology
4525 Third Ave. SE, Ste. 200
Lacy, WA 98503
www.wwctc.com
360-754-3934

Yale University Integrative Medicine
Center – Griffin Hospital
350 Seymour Ave.
Derby, CT 06418
www.imc-griffin.org
203-732-1370

Zakim Center for Integrated Therapies
at Dana-Farber Cancer Institute
44 Binney St.
Shields Warren Bldg. #560
Boston, MA 02115
www.dana-farber.org/pat/support/
zakim
617-632-3322

Appendix B

The following list of integrative oncology related foundations is not exhaustive, but rather a representation of foundations supporting complementary cancer treatment readily available at the time of publication. Criteria for the listing include the provision of grants and allocations exclusively to the advancement of integrative oncology and CAM therapies. The author assumes no responsibility for the accuracy or credibility of the organizations. Updates to this list may be obtained at and submitted to www.cancerchoices.org.

Connie Thompson Foundation
102 Farr Shores Cove
Hot Springs, AR 71913
www.cancerchoices.org
501-617-5559

Foundation for Integrative Oncology (supports San Francisco Bay area only)
P.O. Box 5031
Lakespur, CA 94977
www.complementarycancercare.org
415-721-9818

Helen Moss Breast Cancer Research Foundation
9619 Lakeshore Blvd.
Bratenahl, OH 44108
www.helenmoss.org
216-851-1417

Institute for Integrative Cancer Research and Education
1800 Sherman, Suite 350
Evanston, IL 60201
www.blockmd.com/foundation
847-492-3040

Institute of East West Medicine
102 E. 30th St.
New York, NY 10016
www.eastwestmed.org
212-683-1083

Linus Pauling Institute – Oregon State University
850 SW 35th St.
Corvallis, OR 97333
www.lpi.oregonstate.edu
800-354-7281

Appendix C

STATISTICS TO REMEMBER

The following statistics are provided as quick reference for use in remembering and articulating key data from this book. Sources for the data are cited in the book and are available in the reference section.

- Over 1500 cancer victims die each day from the disease. That is over 560,000 cancer deaths per year.

- The annual rate of death from cancer is 181 per 100,000. That rate has decreased only 9% in the last 35 years (increased 8% to 1990, then decreased 16% to 2006).

- Since the war on cancer was declared by the president in 1971, Americans have spent over $200 billion to wage the war.

- Over 18 million people have died of cancer since 1971. That is 16 times more cancer deaths than the number of deaths from all of our nation's wars combined.

- Of all cancer research funding in the U. S., only about 1% is allocated to CAM or the advancement of integrative oncology.

- Visits by Americans to CAM providers far exceed the number of visits to primary care physicians.

- The amount Americans spend on CAM therapies is about the same as is spent on all physician services.

- Medical care comprises 17% of America's Gross Domestic Product. That is $2.4 trillion, or $7,900 for every man, woman, and child.

- In America, 140,000 people die each year from FDA approved drugs.

- Drug makers employ about 3,000 lobbyists at the federal level.

- Direct medical costs of all cancer health expenditures in America total $93 billion each year.

- It takes an average of about 12 years and costs over $800 million to process one drug through America's new medicines approval system.

REFERENCES

American Cancer Society. 2007. "Society Report Describes Historic Drop in Cancer Deaths." Retrieved from www.cancer.org.

——. 2007. "Combined Financial Statement, 2007." Retrieved from www.cancer.org.

——. 2008. "Annual Report to the Nation on the Status of Cancer, 1975-2005." (Nov. 20).

——. 2009. "Annual Report, 2008," Retrieved from www.cancer.org.

——. 2009. *Costs of Cancer*. Retrieved from www.cancer.org.

The Associated Press. 2007. "Texas Plans to Invest Billions for Cancer Research" *The Sentinel-Record*. (Jan. 24).

Biopharmaceutical Research Inc. 2009. "From the Discovery Lab to the Clinic and Pharmacy." Retrieved from www.bripharm.com.

The Boston Globe. 2007. "Critics Blast Slow Progress on Cancer." (Dec. 2).

The Bravewell Collaborative. 2009. *Changing the Way Physicians are Educated*. Retrieved from www.bravewell.org.

Britt, Robert R. 2005. "The Odds of Dying." *Live Science*. Retrieved from www.livescience.com.

Bruss, K. Ed. 2000. *American Cancer Society's Guide to Complementary and Alternative Cancer Methods.* American Cancer Society.

BSD Medical. 2008. "Hyperthermia Offers a Beam of Hope amidst Gloomy Progress in Cancer Therapy." Press Release retrieved from www.bsdmedical.com.

The Cancer Nutrition Center. 2007. "Nutrition and Cancer: What is the Connection." Retrieved from www.cancernutrition.com.

CBS News. 2008. "The Kanzius Machine: A Cancer Cure?" *CBS News.* Retrieved from www.cbsnews.com.

Centers for Medicare and Medicaid Services. 2008. National Health Expenditures Forecast Summary and Selected Tables.

Contract Pharma. 2009. "2009 Top 20 Pharmaceutical Companies Report," *Contract Pharma.* Retrieved from www.contractpharma.com.

Cook, M. G. 1980. *Cancer Research.* Vol. 40. P. 1329.

Coosa Valley Technical College. 2007. "History of Radiation Therapy." Retrieved from www.cvtcollege.org.

Davis, D., Herbst, R., Abbruzzese, J. (Eds.). 2008. *Antiangiogenic Cancer Therapy.* Boca Raton, LA.: CRC Press

Dufresne, C. J., Farnworth, E. R. 2008. "A Review of Latest Research Findings on the Health Promotion Properties of Tea." *Journal of Nutrition Biochemistry.* Vol. 12. p. 404.

The Economist. 2004. "The Future of Cancer Treatment, Up Close and Personal." (Oct. 14).

Fortune Magazine. 2004. "Why We're Losing the War on Cancer (and How to Win It)." (Mar. 22)

Griffin, G. Edward. 1997. *World Without Cancer.* California: American Media.

References

Harris Interactive. 2007. "Lynn Payer's *Medicine & Culture* Revisited." Retrieved from www.HarrisInteractive.com.

Hau, D. M. 1990. *International Journal of Oriental Medicine.* Vol. 15. p. 10.

Insure.com. 2009. "Insurance Coverage for Alternative Medicine." Retrieved from www.insure.com.

Jemal, Ahmedin. 2010. "Cancer Statistics." *CA, A Cancer Journal for Clinicians.* Retrieved from www.caonline.amcancersoc.org.

Jie, Y. H. 1984. *Agents Actions.* Vol. 15. p. 386.

Journal of the AMA. 1998. "Incidents of Adverse Drug Reactions in Hospital Patients." Vol. 279, No. 15. (Apr. 15).

Kolde, T. 1996. *Cancer Biotherapy and Radiopharmaceuticals.* Vol. 11. p.273.

Komen for the Cure. 2007. Retrieved from www.komen.org.

Kuttan, R. 1985. *Cancer Letters.* Vol. 29. p. 197.

———. 1987. *Tumori.* Vol. 73. p. 29.

LeBon, A. M. 1992. *Chemical Biological Interactions.* Vol. 83.

Li, X. 1991. *Journal of Tongji Medical University.* Vol. 11. p. 73.

The Light Party. 2008. "Accidental Deaths from Prescription Drugs," Retrieved from www.lightparty.com.

Ludwig Institute for Cancer Research. 2010. "Fact Sheet." Retrieved from www.licr.org.

Marsh, C.L. 1987. *Journal of Urology.* Vol. 137. p. 359.

Mary. 2006. American Cancer Society email message to author.

Medscape Medical News. 2007. "Cancer Survival Rates Improving Across Europe, But Still Lagging Behind United States." Retrieved from www.medscape.com.

Micksche, M. 1978. *Onkologie*, Vol. 1, p. 57.

Moss, Ralph. 2009. "A victory for Hyperthermia in Bladder Cancer." *Cancer Decisions*. Retrieved from www.cancerdecisions.com.

The National Academy of Sciences. 2005. "Complementary and Alternative Medicine in the United States." p. 35.

National Audit Office, London. 2008. "International Health Comparisons, 2003."

National Center for Health Statistics. 2008. "Actual Number of Cancer Deaths." Retrieved from www.cdc.gov.

NCI. 2008. "FY 2010 Budget." Retrieved from www.plan.cancer.gov.

———. 2008. "Surveillance Epidemiology and End Results (SEER)." Retrieved from www.seer.cancer.gov.

———. 2008. *Annual Report to the Nation on the Status of Cancer, 1975-2005.* Journal of the National Cancer Institute.

———. 2008. "Understanding Cancer Series: Gene Testing." *NCI Cancer Topics*. Retrieved from www.cancer.gov.

———. 2008. "Vaccine Treats Breast Tumors in Mice." *NCI Cancer Bulletin.* (Apr. 1).

———. 2008. "Herbal Therapy for Brain Cancer." *NCI Cancer Bulletin,* (Apr. 15).

———. 2008. "Vitamin C Injections Slow Tumor Growth in Mice." *NCI Cancer Bulletin.* (Aug. 19).

———. 2009. "2009 Fact Book." Retrieved from www.obf.cancer.gov.

References

Oluwadamilola Olaku, MD, et.al. 2005. *Survey of Cancer Researchers and Practitioners Regarding Complementary and Alternative Medicine.* Retrieved from www.integrativeonc.org.

Ornish, Dean, MD. 2005. *Lifestyle Changes.* Sausalito, CA: Preventive Medicine Research Institute.

Park, C. H. 1980. *Cancer Research.* Vol. 40, p.1062.

Payer, Lynn. 1988. *Medicine and Culture: Varieties of Treatment in the United States, England, West Germany, and France.* New York: Holt.

Poydock, M. E. 1991. *American Journal of Clinical Nutrition.* Vol. 54, p. 1261S.

PR Web Press Release Newswire. 2008. Retrieved from www.prweb.com.

President Richard M. Nixon Speech. "The State of the Union." (Jan. 22).

Public Integrity. 2008. "Drug Lobby Second to None," *Special Report.* Retrieved from www.publicintegrity.org.

———. 2008. "How the Pharmaceutical Industry Gets Its Way in Washington." *Special Report.* Retrieved from www.publicintegrity.org.

———. 2008. "Drug Makers' Dime Funds Congressional Travel." *Power Trips.* Retrieved from www.publicintegrity.org.

Quillin, P. PhD. 1998. *Beating Cancer with Nutrition.* Tulsa, OK.: Nutrition Times Press

Rabin, R. C. 2008. "Lengthy Fall in U.S. Cancer Rates a First." *The New York Times.* (Nov. 25)

Sampson, David. 2010. American Cancer Society (Media). "CAM Allocation." ACS email to the author.

Shea. 2010. National Cancer Institute telephone conversation with author.

Shklar, G. 1987. *Journal of the National Cancer Institute.* Vol. 78, p. 987.

Steve. 2008. "Re: SEER.cancer.gov. comment: Mortality Rates." NCI Email to the author.

Stich, H. F. 1991. *American Journal of Clinical Nutrition.* Vol. 53. p. 298S.

Stobbe, M. 2008. 1 in 9 U.S. Kids Use Alternative Medicine. *The Sentinel-Record.* (Dec. 16).

The Washington Post. 2008. "Frankincense Provides Relief for Osteoarthritis." (Jul. 30).

USA Today. 1998. "Drug Reactions Kill 100,000 Patients a Year." (Apr. 15).

U.S. Department of Veterans Affairs. 2009. *Fact Sheet: America's Wars.* Retrieved from www.va.gov.

U.S. News. 2010. "What Is the Actual Number of Persons without Health Insurance?" Retrieved from www.usnews.com.

Wargovich, M. J. 1992. *Cancer Letters.* Vol. 64. p. 39.

Wattenberg, L. 1970. *Cancer Research.* Vol. 30. p. 1922.

Werbach, M. 1994. *Botanical Influences on Illness.* p. 30. Tarzana, CA.: Third Line Press

Wikipedia. 2007. "William Stewart Halsted," and "Radical Mastectomy." Retrieved from www.wikipedia.org

Wood, L. 1985. "Possible Prevention of Adriamiacin-induced Alopecia by Tocopherol." *New England Journal of Medicine.* 312-1060.

World Health Organization. 2008. "Health Statistics and Health Information Systems." Retrieved from www.who.int.

INDEX

Medicine and Culture 54, 267
meditation xiii, 8, 9, 25, 30, 135,
    143, 197, 241
mega dose vitamins 8, 9
Memorial Sloan-Kettering Cancer
    Center 22, 105, 257
Merck 173, 174
metastasis 49, 75, 111–113
metastasize 38, 92, 108, 109,
    111–113, 150
metastasized tumors 111
Michigan State University 200
milk thistle 82
mind-body therapy 141–143, 197
Mitchell, John 172
Mitomycin-C 94
Moertel, Dr. Charles 115, 116
monoclonal antibodies xii, 91, 92
monoclonal antibody therapy 91
monopolistic 166, 175, 180
Monsanto Chemical 168
mortality rate 17, 26, 60, 61, 165,
    166, 173, 229, 268
mustard gas 43

N

Nahin, Richard 68
nanoparticles 98, 99, 100
National Academy of Sciences 30,
    76, 218, 266
National Cancer Act 18, 21
National Cancer Institute (NCI) 8,
    16, 17, 28, 52, 94, 97, 115, 163,
    266, 267
National Center for Complementary
    and Alternative Medicine
    (NCCAM) 3, 24, 68

National Center for Epidemiology,
    Health Surveillance, and
    Promotion 56
National Institutes of Health (NIH)
    3, 18, 75, 76, 115, 163
National Polytechnic Institute 121
Natural Killer cells 120
Natural Killer (NK) cell 83
natural medicine 119, 120, 165,
    167, 178, 182, 209, 220
Natural Solutions Magazine 140
Naturemed Integrative Medicine
    257
naturopathic 8, 69, 79, 157, 220
NCI Cancer Bulletin 76, 80, 266
New Again 248
New England Journal of Medicine
    78, 115, 268
Newman, Robert, Ph.D 70
New York Academy of Sciences 72
niacin 73
Niederhuber, John 61
Nivenny, Dr. Hans 152
Nixon, President Richard xii, 3, 16,
    18, 21, 171, 217, 267
non-pharmacological 8, 9, 116, 163,
    176, 178
North American Association of
    Central Cancer Registries 60
Novartis 173, 174
nutrition xii, xiii, 4, 25, 45, 62, 67,
    69–71, 74, 76, 83, 84, 86, 87,
    96, 108, 119, 120, 128, 133, 135,
    141, 142, 151, 153, 197, 219,
    243, 264, 267, 268

O

Oasis of Hope Hospital vi, 107

W

Warner-Lambert Pharmaceutical
172
Washington University-St. Louis
200
Wentz, Dr. Myron 118, 120
western medicine xii, 8
Western Washington Oncology 258
Whatley, Franklin 149, 155
What to Eat if You Have Cancer 83
white blood cells 38, 42, 43, 46, 47,
93, 121
White, Maria Claudia vi, 139–149,
158
WHO 164
window of efficacy for vitamins 73
Women's Primary Care/Integ. Med
200
World War II xii, 43, 58, 62, 168,
169, 183, 228, 231
worship 108, 135, 153
WWI 183

Y

Yale University 70, 124, 200, 258

Z

Zakim Center for Integrated
Therapies 258
zinc 83

BUY A SHARE OF THE FUTURE IN YOUR COMMUNITY

These certificates make great holiday, graduation and birthday gifts that can be personalized with the recipient's name. The cost of one S.H.A.R.E. or one square foot is $54.17. The personalized certificate is suitable for framing and will state the number of shares purchased and the amount of each share, as well as the recipient's name. The home that you participate in "building" will last for many years and will continue to grow in value.

Here is a sample SHARE certificate:

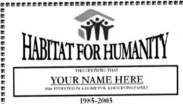

HABITAT FOR HUMANITY

THIS CERTIFIES THAT
YOUR NAME HERE
HAS INVESTED IN A HOME FOR A DESERVING FAMILY

1985-2005
TWENTY YEARS OF BUILDING FUTURES IN OUR
COMMUNITY ONE HOME AT A TIME

1200 SQUARE FOOT HOUSE @ $65,000 = $54.17 PER SQUARE FOOT
This certificate represents a tax deductible donation. It has no cash value.

YES, I WOULD LIKE TO HELP!

I support the work that Habitat for Humanity does and I want to be part of the excitement! As a donor, I will receive periodic updates on your construction activities but, more importantly, I know my gift will help a family in our community realize the dream of homeownership. **I would like to SHARE in your efforts against substandard housing in my community!** *(Please print below)*

PLEASE SEND ME _____ SHARES at $54.17 EACH = $ $_____

In Honor Of: _____

Occasion: (Circle One) HOLIDAY   BIRTHDAY   ANNIVERSARY

OTHER: _____

Address of Recipient: _____

Gift From: _____ *Donor Address:* _____

Donor Email: _____

I AM ENCLOSING A CHECK FOR $ $_____ PAYABLE TO HABITAT FOR HUMANITY OR PLEASE CHARGE MY VISA OR MASTERCARD *(CIRCLE ONE)*

Card Number _____ Expiration Date: _____

Name as it appears on Credit Card _____ Charge Amount $ _____

Signature _____

Billing Address _____

Telephone # Day _____ Eve _____

PLEASE NOTE: Your contribution is tax-deductible to the fullest extent allowed by law.
Habitat for Humanity • P.O. Box 1443 • Newport News, VA 23601 • 757-596-5553
www.HelpHabitatforHumanity.org

LaVergne, TN USA
28 December 2010
210369LV00006B/7/P